World Health Organization
Regional Office for Europe
Copenhagen

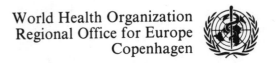

Priority research
for
health for all

European Health for All Series, No. 3

ICP/RPD 110
Text editing by: M.S. Burgher

ISBN 92 890 1054 1

PRINTED IN ENGLAND

CONTENTS

Preface

This book is the third in the new European Health for All Series. The first[a] set out the European policy on health for all. The second[b] dealt with research policy; this companion publication moves from policy to practice, pointing out the topics and methods of research needed to help achieve health for all in the European Region.

History shows an impressive record of contributions by research to the improvement of health. The knowledge supplied by the research community has been one of the most valuable tools in the struggle against disease, disability and death. Researchers feel justifiable pride in their past and present work. With its remarkable track record, vast resources and sense of responsibility to society, the European research community will want to grasp the exciting new opportunity detailed in this book: the chance to contribute to health for all and thereby to expand and develop the field of research.

The Member States of the WHO European Region have pledged to reach the goal of health for all by achieving the 38 regional targets. Action, however, requires knowledge, both existing information and that yet to be discovered. Research can generate the knowledge

---

[a] *Targets for health for all.* Copenhagen, WHO Regional Office for Europe, 1985 (European Health for All Series, No. 1).

[b] *Research policies for health for all.* Copenhagen, WHO Regional Office for Europe, 1988 (European Health for All Series, No. 2).

required; the role of the research community in the health for all movement is thus a vital one. The targets call for specific improvements in health. What, specifically, are the implications of the targets for research?

The European Advisory Committee on Health Research carefully analysed each of the targets. This book is the result of the regional analysis: a framework that countries can use to set their own priorities for research for health for all. The publication sets out five overriding themes of priority research in the Region. It discusses in practical terms the topics and methods of research needed to achieve each target, and the resulting opportunities for the research community.

Within these pages is an array of fascinating topics for research that is highly likely to contribute to the attainment of health for all. By choosing the topics that meet their needs, countries and scientists can discover vital new knowledge and determine how to use existing knowledge more effectively. The priority research described here builds on the scientific successes of the past and the endeavours of the present; it offers the European scientific community the chance to work in new areas and with new colleagues, using research to build health for all.

J.E. Asvall
WHO Regional Director
for Europe

Introduction

Knowledge is essential to transform a policy into a reality and research is the most powerful tool for generating this knowledge. Research — most often basic biomedical work on topics chosen by the investigators themselves — has supplied the knowledge behind the greatest victories in the fight against disease, disability and death. Such research is still undeniably valuable.

Health for all through research

Nevertheless, the WHO Regional Office for Europe and the Member States of the Region are asking for a fundamental change in research. They ask that this tool be used more effectively than ever before, to reach a specific goal: health for all. They ask that policy-makers and the research community of each country work together to provide the knowledge needed to reach this goal, by building and using research strategies suited to their special needs.

Policy-makers and the research community in each Member State of the Region should cooperate to determine what research is most important, according to their own priorities, perform the studies and use the results to improve health. By taking up this challenge both groups will not just work more effectively; they will also make a better future for themselves and for society by helping to achieve health for all.

Health for all — global, regional and in countries — is the most ambitious health policy ever set. The Member States of WHO have chosen a far-reaching goal: health for all people by the year 2000.

What health for all means

1

At the heart of the health for all movement is a new look at health with a broader perspective. Health remains the goal of health policies and health care systems, but it has a wider definition. The Member States have pledged to attain for their people more than a reduction in disease and disability. They are working for a positive kind of health: a state of complete physical, mental and social wellbeing. Reaching such a goal requires a wider view of the factors that affect health, encompassing something more than the physical problems of individual people. This view must examine the ways in which factors in society and in the environment affect people's health. A policy for health for all thus requires positive health to be built in new ways and new settings, by new combinations of people, in addition to the methods and means used successfully in the past.

The European Member States have taken the first steps towards their revolutionary goal. Through their representatives in the Regional Committee for Europe, the parliament of the Regional Office, they adopted 38 regional targets as concrete goals to work towards, and 65 regional indicators by which to measure their progress.[a] Briefly put, the targets describe how present conditions must be changed to reach health for all.

The 38 regional targets

The regional targets are not legal bonds on any Member State. They form a flexible framework that the political authorities, professional groups and general public of each nation can use to build their own targets, policies and programmes for health for all.

The targets have been carefully designed, and they fit as closely together as the blocks of stone that compose a pyramid. Each rests on the support of others and dovetails neatly with its neighbours. The apex of the pyramid is equity (target 1), to be attained by reducing present inequalities in health between and within countries.

The targets can be divided into three closely related groups, according to their purposes and their dates of completion. Fig. 1 illustrates this relationship.

---

[a] *Targets for health for all.* Copenhagen, WHO Regional Office for Europe, 1985 (European Health for All Series, No. 1).

2

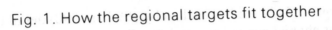

Fig. 1. How the regional targets fit together

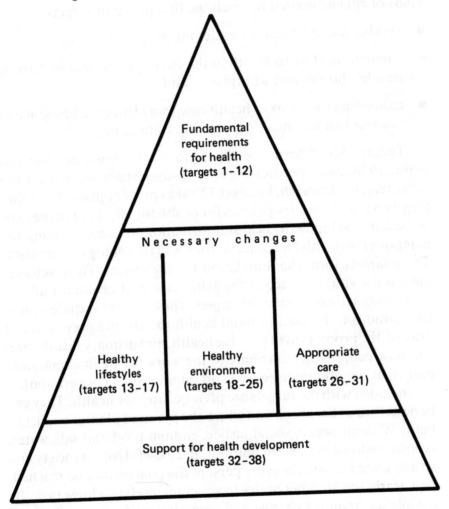

Fundamental
requirements
for health
(targets 1–12)

Necessary changes

Healthy
lifestyles
(targets 13–17)

Healthy
environment
(targets 18–25)

Appropriate
care
(targets 26–31)

Support for health development
(targets 32–38)

Targets 1–12 (to be achieved by the year 2000) are the fundamental requirements for health. These include equity, a longer and better life for all, and reductions in deaths from certain causes. Their achievement will mean that health for all is a reality.

3

Targets 13–31 (to be reached by 1995 or 1990) detail the three kinds of change needed to reach the first group of targets:

- making healthy lifestyles easier for people to choose;

- eliminating risks to health in the environment and improving people's homes and workplaces; and

- redirecting the focus of health care away from the hospital and towards primary health care in the community.

Targets 32–38 form the third group and must be achieved before 1990. Each specifies one kind of support needed to reach the other targets. Research, in target 32, takes pride of place. The other targets concern country policies for health for all, the management of health development, health information systems, training for manpower in health and other sectors, and technology assessment. These targets form the foundation for the others. Their achievement is the vital first step in the achievement of health for all.

Common themes unite the targets. These themes include equity, the methods to be used to build health for all (the prevention of disease, the promotion of positive health, and primary health care) and how people can contribute to the work (through community participation, and intersectoral and international cooperation).

Included with the targets are prerequisites for health. They can be described as the ground on which the pyramid of targets must be built. Without peace, social justice, enough food and safe water, adequate education, decent housing, and a useful role in society and an adequate income for every person, the goal cannot be reached.

Clearly the Member States have set themselves a huge task. Its completion requires change and commitment from people in all sectors of society in every Member State. People must discover how their work affects health and work actively with others for health for all. Five groups of people have rights to and responsibilities in health for all; health authorities at all levels (including policy-makers and administrators), health professionals of all kinds (including the research community), the people, sectors other than health, and international organizations.

This book sets out topics for research for health for all that should appeal to members of the second group. A related publication[a] discusses the responsibilities of and opportunities that both the research community and policy-makers can find in working together for health for all.

The targets are to be achieved within a very short time (2–12 years). Action for health for all, based on knowledge, is plainly needed. Part of this knowledge already exists, and health for all would not be so far away if it were used. New knowledge is also needed. How to acquire and apply knowlege for health for all is a question that demands a response.

The Regional Committee's answer is target 32.

The answer:
research strategies

Before 1990, all Member States should have formulated research strategies to stimulate investigations which improve the application and expansion of knowledge needed to support their health for all developments.

This target can be achieved if Member States establish machinery to ensure the effective application of new knowledge in the development of health policies and programmes; determine what gaps there are in the knowledge needed to support the strategy of health for all and set research priorities accordingly; ensure a balanced representation of all academic disciplines relevant to health and of providers and users of health services as well as health policy-makers, in the planning and coordinating of research for health for all and make the research community an active contributor to the development of health for all; stimulate relevant multidisciplinary research; and allocate sufficient resources to conduct the research needed, giving preference to aspects that have not received the support they deserve.

Target 32.
Research and
health for all

---

[a] *Research policies for health for all.* Copenhagen, WHO Regional Office for Europe, 1988 (European Health for All Series, No. 2).

In other words, the Member States of the Region have agreed that research strategies, resulting in guided research directed at specific goals, will ensure that the knowledge needed to attain health for all is provided and used well.

The targets cover fields of activity that are fundamental to public health but new subjects for country policies and health research. The structure of the targets suggests six broad tasks:

- describing every aspect of the health of the population so that progress towards the targets can be monitored (target 32);

- finding out what biological factors determine health (targets 1–12);

- assessing the part that lifestyles play in maintaining or endangering health (targets 13–17);

- studying the ways in which the physical, biological and social environment (including the basic prerequisites for health) determine the health of individuals and populations (targets 13–25);

- developing effective and efficient methods of providing people with appropriate care (targets 26–31); and

- improving policy-making, planning and management in programmes for health for all (targets 32–38).

To provide the necessary knowledge, health research must venture for the first time into fields that lie outside its traditional domain, the health and related sciences. To succeed, health researchers must seek cooperation with people in all the disciplines that can contribute the expert knowledge necessary. This will mainly involve the biomedical, behavioural and social sciences, although questions will also arise that will require answers from, for example, engineers, architects and other specialists.

Researchers working for health for all will take their expertise into new, unfamiliar areas and work with new colleagues in new ways. The research community has the chance not only to continue basic research for health but also, through goal-directed research, to take part directly in making and carrying out health and research policies. The research community can thus help to decide the future of its own profession by contributing to health for all.

When adopting the targets in 1984, the Regional Committee asked the European Advisory Committee on Health Research (EACHR) to help create a regional strategy for research for health for all. The EACHR (16 experts on different kinds of research, health administration, and research policies and administration) had two tasks: to advise the Regional Office for Europe on its regional policy on research for health for all, and to analyse each of the regional targets, to discover what kinds of research were most needed. In both tasks, the EACHR worked to meet three needs.

What research is needed?

The first was flexibility. Strategies for health for all must be carried out in all 32 Member States of the European Region, an area bounded by Norway in the north, Israel and Turkey in the south-east, the USSR in the east, Iceland in the north-west and Portugal in the south-west. All these countries have widely different patterns of mortality and morbidity, health care systems and research capacities. All must determine their own priorities and the regional research strategy must provide them with a framework and a guide for their own strategies.

The time frame for completing priority research had to be equally flexible. The completion dates set for the regional targets — some as early as 1990 — are far too restrictive to be applied to research. The regional strategy must point out areas of research that will contribute to achieving the targets, even if applicable results cannot be produced within such narrow time limits. A flexible time frame is particularly necessary to the opening of new areas of investigation.

Second, the regional strategy, and the analysis of the targets in particular, had to make specific recommendations for priority research to attain the targets. The EACHR therefore analysed the targets one by one, along with the Regional Committee's discussion of and suggestions for attaining them.

The third requirement was participation. Individual scientists, the scientific community, and national and international research bodies were all needed to take part in developing the regional strategy from the outset. They were to point out gaps in knowledge and the resulting needs for research. They were also to suggest, discuss and agree on both the research projects required and the timing of their implementation.

The work of the EACHR was considered by the Regional Committee, the Regional Health Development Advisory Council, the Consultative Group on Programme Development (15 senior health administrators who advise the WHO Regional Director for Europe on the regional programme), ministries of health, ministries responsible for science and technology, medical research councils, and by members of the research community, before it gained final approval from the Regional Committee at its thirty-seventh session in 1987. This book is one of the results.

Research strategies for Member States

Target 32 requests Member States to make research strategies to support their progress towards health for all. Like the regional targets, the regional research strategy outlined here is an opportunity, not a prescription that all countries must follow to the letter. It should inspire European countries to develop research strategies that meet their priorities and needs by offering a framework on which they can construct their own research policies and projects. It is also designed to help countries to attain regional and country targets by translating them into concrete research recommendations, by enlisting the support of the research community for health for all, by guiding the allocation of research resources in Member States, and by stimulating all sectors to include health for all in their research policies. Finally, the regional strategy will guide the research activities of the Regional Office.

The regional strategy for research for health for all has three parts:

- an analysis of the most important research needs arising from the targets;

- a research policy that sets criteria for choosing research topics of high priority, and spells out the material and human resources needed and ways to ensure that they are provided; and

- a plan to promote and carry out the strategy.

Country strategies could have the same components.

This book contains the first part of the regional strategy. Here the regional targets are analysed, singly and in groups, for their research implications. Although specific research needs will vary from country to country, the targets themselves hint strongly at the kinds of research most useful in their achievement. Research policies and a plan for promoting them are discussed in the related publication, *Research policies for health for all.*

The roles of the scientific community and health authorities, policy-makers and administrators cannot be separated for discussion as easily as the parts of a research strategy. While the scientific community is likely to be most interested in this book and health authorities and the people who make health policy will be most concerned with the companion publication, their roles are closely intertwined. As proof of the close relationship between both the subjects of and the audiences for the two books, the publications have an introduction and first chapter in common.

Just as community participation is a cornerstone of health for all, so cooperation between and within both groups is essential to the success of strategies for research for health for all. An effective strategy demands that policy-makers and researchers help each other to fulfil their complementary roles. Policy-makers should point out important topics for research. Researchers should not only study these, but advise policy-makers on their choices and help to make both research policy and plans for using the knowledge gained. Policy-makers should then use these findings to plan and run health care systems and services. Finally, researchers should evaluate the success of the whole strategy.

By working together within the regional and country research strategies, policy-makers and the research community can produce not only vital knowledge for health for all but also the kind of intersectoral collaboration that will help to make it a reality.

The regional analysis: a framework for setting priorities

This regional analysis of the targets for health for all identifies the areas of research needed to attain them. Just as health for all calls upon the scientific community to take part in research policy, so policy-makers can profit from the discussion of priority areas of research. While the regional analysis displays an inventory of tempting opportunities to the scientific community, it also carries implications for research policy by suggesting priorities among the different topics. These priorities will be particularly interesting to the people in charge of policy on health research at country level. The regional analysis is a starting point from which researchers and makers of country policies on research for health for all can take their first step: choosing their own priorities.

In analysing each of the 38 regional targets, the European Advisory Committee on Health Research worked to stimulate research of priority in the struggle to achieve regional and country targets, not all possible research related to health. The members of the Committee tried to choose research topics that are:

Choosing priority areas for research

● highly likely to contribute to the attainment of the regional targets (preferably but not exclusively within the time frame suggested by the Regional Committee);

- closely linked to the Regional Committee's suggested solutions for attainment,[a] although other options will be pursued;

- likely to yield results that can be translated into health policy and action; and

- unfortunately, likely to be neglected otherwise, despite their importance.

The Member States themselves pinpointed gaps in knowledge and problems in achieving the targets in the first of their triennial evaluations of their progress towards health for all.[b]

Common themes The regional targets share common themes, vital elements of their success: equity, disease prevention, health promotion, primary health care, community participation, and intersectoral and international cooperation. Similar themes run through research for health for all. They include three areas of research:

— health policy and organizational behaviour

— inequities

— community participation and intersectoral collaboration

and two essential tools:

— better information systems and indicators for the targets

— international comparative studies.

---

[a] Solutions for attaining the targets are thoroughly discussed in *Targets for health for all* (Copenhagen, WHO Regional Office for Europe, 1985 (European Health for All Series, No. 1)).

[b] *Evaluation of the strategy for health for all by the year 2000. Seventh report on the world health situation. Vol. 5: European Region.* Copenhagen, WHO Regional Office for Europe, 1986.

Naturally, many concrete research questions can touch several themes. The importance of the themes will, of course, vary from country to country.

Research on health policy and organizational behaviour is an overriding priority for four main reasons.

First, although enough information is already available to take firm action on many targets, nothing is being done. Research on implementation is therefore needed. Most of the problems of, obstacles to and constraints on implementation can be understood by applying the concepts and methods of such disciplines as political science, sociology, social policy and management science. In addition, policy formulation should be systematically scrutinized as a social process. This is a difficult area of study. In implementation analysis in particular, the researcher must deal with vested interests and the inevitable problems arising from the definitions used. Researchers must also have the courage not only to recognize that no further information is needed but to tell policy-makers that the time has come for action.

Second, current health care systems do not function as well as they should. In many important areas, current services are based on conventional wisdom rather than hard scientific evidence. Health systems research and evaluative research can help to show the best way to deliver services. Technology assessment will allow people to choose technology of proven safety, efficiency, effectiveness and acceptability. Finally, quality assurance will see that high standards of care are met.

Third, the regional targets detail changes in the organization of health care systems, and emphasize community participation in and consumer satisfaction with health services as keys to health for all. The targets call for several far-reaching structural changes. These include: a shift of emphasis from the hospital to primary health care as the focus of health care, more teamwork among health personnel, more systematic mechanisms for quality assurance and technology assessment, the promotion of more effective community participation, the encouragement of mutual-aid groups, and the introduction of systematic planning for research. Such changes must be founded on knowledge of the conditions, constraints and consequences of organizational development.

Fourth, the direction of health research needs to be scrutinized. Researchers are usually more interested in providing better means to reach the goals of social and health policies than in questioning these goals. Now may be the time to make a critical analysis of the goals of research, particularly research on health systems. Such work often focuses more on the quality, accessibility and cost-efficiency of services and systems than on their effects on health, acceptability, and ethical and political desirability.

Priority research on health policy and organizational behaviour should address:

- the relationship between overall social policy goals, health policy and people's health;

- influences on the design and implementation of health policy;

- the means of carrying out health policy and the priority ranking of health policy goals;

- the role of other sectors in health care;

- the relationship between official and unofficial (professional and lay) care systems and between public and private care sectors;

- the organizational and administrative structures of central, regional and local health care;

- the cost–benefit ratio, cost-efficiency and cost-effectiveness of new and established health services; and

- the quality of care.

Research on inequities
    Target 1 deals with equity in health. This is no accident; raising the overall level of health and increasing equity are the two basic goals of health care. People may suffer from inequities because of their social status or class, sex, ethnic group or geographic location. Despite the

14

position of equity as the pinnacle of the targets, establishing a reliable picture of equity within and between countries will be very difficult until they improve their information base on this critical issue.

Research on equity should include:

- defining concepts and creating indicators to measure inequities in health;
- gaining a better understanding of the factors and mechanisms that create and maintain inequities; and
- studying policies and evaluating programmes to reduce health inequities.

Community participation and intersectoral collaboration, themes of the regional targets, are two of the cornerstones of all work for health for all. Relatively little is known, however, about how they have been organized. Less is known about their effects on the cost, effectiveness, quality and acceptability of health policies and services. Even the idea of community participation is poorly defined. Studies on such questions are urgently needed. Determining the role of community participation in primary health care is particularly important.

Research on community participation and intersectoral collaboration

Better information is so urgently needed that one of the targets is devoted to it. Today's information systems do not provide the kinds of information necessary to achieve the targets or to measure progress towards achieving them. Weaknesses can be found in: the definition of concepts of and boundaries between sectors of health care, and the availability, reliability and interpretation of data. It is also difficult to disaggregate data in a way that makes them relevant to various population, administrative and geographical groups. Finally, the length, techniques and coverage of reporting vary among countries.

Need for better information

Current data also say very little about such problems in health care as the quality of life, overtreatment, iatrogenic disease, the feelings of alienation in patients and their families, the unwanted extension of life, or the emotional and financial costs of illness to the family. Further, present information systems are not well suited to assessing equity.

This problem calls for two remedies: the development of better information systems, and, within these, the development of better indicators for evaluating progress.

Research is needed to standardize procedures for data collection and to assess the cost-effectiveness of collecting new data. A balance must also be struck between the legitimate needs of policy-makers and researchers for information and the protection of patients' rights to privacy and confidentiality.

Health information systems.   Most health information systems have been designed to collect administrative data. They are often simple "head counts" showing, for example, how much money has been spent or how many surgical operations have been performed.

The usefulness of the information collected can be increased in two ways. First, the value of a single item of data can be enhanced by making it more detailed and precise or by adding modifiers to derive secondary data. For example, the severity of conditions could be recorded along with diagnoses or a price tag or estimate could be attached to the record of each service used. Cost-analysis or time-and-motion studies may be needed to obtain such modifiers. Second, several items of data can be combined in various ways to provide more meaningful information.

Looking at the relationships between data will produce useful information for health planning, evaluation and health service research. More must be known than the total number of services produced; research must reveal the impact of care on people's health — not just the number of patients discharged but their satisfaction with their care. Other neglected areas are the safety and acceptability of procedures to patients and the cost-effectiveness of services. Information systems should also allow researchers to identify and analyse differences in health care practices.

Indicators.   Developing a standard system of collecting information is one of the most pressing needs in research for health for all. This system should be applied to all the kinds of data that are relevant to achieving the targets but either unavailable at present or interpreted differently from country to country. Research must focus on the types of data that should be collected; how to define, store, retrieve and evaluate them; and what kinds of feedback mechanism must be established to monitor specific programmes.

New indicators of health need to be developed or existing ones must be improved in several areas.[a] Equity is perhaps the most important, but problems that cross national boundaries also deserve special attention. Most indicators on these issues are qualitative; quantitative indicators should complement them whenever possible. The possibilities for disaggregating data in a meaningful way should be increased. The variables used in the disaggregation should have clear, standard definitions.

New or better indicators are also needed to assess:

- the consumer's view of health care needs;
- early changes in biological systems caused by long-term, low-dose exposure to environmental agents;
- the effectiveness of health care services (results, quality of care, client satisfaction);
- the costs and efficiency of services;
- community participation in health care;
- health behaviour and positive health; and
- the evaluation of health systems development (through the use of "tracers").

The targets call for many profound changes. Such reforms can be risky and costly ventures. The political risks may be great because

International comparative studies

---

[a] A revision of the regional indicators has been endorsed by the Regional Committee for Europe: *Revised list of indicators and procedure for monitoring progress towards health for all in the European Region (1987–1988)* (Copenhagen, WHO Regional Office for Europe, 1987 (unpublished document EUR/RC37/8 Rev.1)).

the outcome cannot always be guaranteed. Policy-makers may want to know about the experience of other countries, particularly if the countries are engaged in similar activities. Such information is often difficult to obtain. It may not be be collected systematically; many variables of interest to other countries may be overlooked. Finally, the information may be unavailable simply because of language barriers or because it is scattered throughout the system.

International comparative studies can help to solve these problems. They can give better insights into many aspects of progress towards health for all than studies conducted within a single country. They are particularly useful in working for appropriate care. Traditions in care and the organization of health services can often be better evaluated when contrasted with those of other countries, where their development has taken a different direction.

Much can be learned from an analysis of the strengths and weaknesses of different countries' approaches to organizing health care. Studies based on rigorous scientific research designs, however, not only are very expensive but also yield results that may be difficult to use. Fortunately, relatively simple and inexpensive descriptive studies may be wholly sufficient for decision-making.

Regular international health surveys might be another solution to the problems of method and expense. The surveys could be carried out in connection with or as a complement to the triennial regional evaluations of progress towards health for all, to avoid duplication of work. To minimize costs and lighten the burden on countries of collecting data, health surveys could cover a sample of Member States and their populations. Although each survey should include certain basic measurements, to enable trends to be assessed, it should also have its own specific focus. Each country should use similar definitions and standardized measurements, to produce comparable results.

International collaborative studies are needed:

- to collate, compare and disseminate the information available in different countries on the strengths and weaknesses of

18

various approaches to providing health services and on many other variables related to the regional targets;

- to carry out truly comparative research according to a common protocol, to study most of the areas related to achieving the regional targets, particularly the area of health policy; and

- to provide models for developing health services.

At the beginning of this book, the 38 regional targets were compared to a pyramid (Fig. 1) because the attainment of each will result from or lead to the attainment of others. Further, the structure they form will lead to a peak of achievement: equity in health. Like architects explaining a design, people explaining the targets begin at the top. They start by discussing the great goal and the other targets that form the 12 fundamental requirements for health for all in Europe. Then they talk about how to get there: through the three groups of necessary changes (healthy lifestyles, a healthy environment and appropriate care). They finish by examining the foundation of the structure, the seven kinds of support needed to make the necessary changes.

Priority research

This is the right way to describe a plan or a completed project. The European Member States, however, are moving from the first to the second position. They have begun the work to achieve the targets, but it is far from over. To build this monument, the countries of Europe are working from the ground up.

For this reason, the regional analysis of the targets begins with the foundation for health for all, the last group of targets, which are to be attained first. This group starts, appropriately enough, with research. The discussion then moves through appropriate care, a healthy environment and healthy lifestyles and ends with the fundamental requirements for health. A chapter is devoted to each group of targets. In each chapter, the targets are analysed first collectively and then one by one, in numerical order.

This order has some interesting features. For example, research grows in importance as the reader moves from group to group. In addition, the reader parallels the journey that researchers and policy-makers will take as they expand their familiar responsibilities to include the new opportunities in health for all.

Some of the landmarks on this journey are familiar. For example, the bulk of health research is already proceeding, most often successfully, towards many of the same goals as the first 12 targets. Why, then, should the Member States and the research community take on the arduous job of working through the targets? The answer lies in the nature of the health for all movement. It is designed not to reject but to build on the successes of the past and present, to reach a more complete kind of health in the future. This means that research will be sharpened and refined and therefore a more effective tool in the work for positive health.

Although research priorities will vary from one country to another, on the basis of the target-by-target analysis, the following summary of overall priorities for each of the five groups of targets may be suggested for Europe as a whole.

Support for health development (targets 32–38)

The last seven targets detail a number of prerequisites for all work to improve health, including research. These requirements must be met to change attitudes and working practices among politicians, health authorities, health personnel, people in other sectors and, above all, the general public. One prerequisite — research strategies (target 32) — is so important that a publication[a] is devoted to it, in addition to the discussion in this book. Another — the need for more detailed, reliable and standardized data for every target (target 34) — is an overriding theme of research for health for all. The other necessary kinds of support are: country health policies committed to the principles of health for all, well trained and motivated health personnel, support from professions outside the health sector, and health care technology that meets people's needs in an effective and an acceptable way.

Increased research is needed for:

— making health policy

---

[a] *Research policies for health for all.* Copenhagen, WHO Regional Office for Europe, 1988 (European Health for All Series, No. 2).

20

— educating health personnel

— assessing health technology.

Health policies based on the principles of health for all can probably best be promoted by a clear demonstration of their advantages: greater effectiveness, efficiency and equity. Therefore, comparative studies, policy research, scenarios and simulation models are needed to determine which health care systems can best meet the goal of improving people's health at minimal cost and in an equitable way.

Ironically, the success of modern health care has created the need to change the education of health personnel. Acute conditions are losing ground to chronic and disabling health problems. The aging of the population will reinforce this trend. The central question here is how to adapt the education of health personnel to the new health needs of the chronically ill, the elderly, the mentally ill and long-term patients. Cultural and recreational needs should be included with needs for medical care. Evaluative research on existing training programmes should compare their objectives (and results) with the new objectives, skills and attitudes required to meet actual health care needs. Different models of education for health personnel should be compared, to point out the curricula and teaching methods most likely to improve health workers' abilities and motivation to provide competent, comprehensive care in the community.

The tendency towards an unchecked expansion of health technology brings a number of evils in its train. The costs of care skyrocket, the providers and users of services are alienated from one another, and patients are treated like objects and lose their responsibility for their own health. The assessment of health technology can control the tendency and fight its unfortunate side effects. Multidisciplinary research is urgently needed at all levels to improve the assessment of health technology.

The work should begin with deciding what technology most needs assessment and setting criteria to make such decisions. Next, the technology selected must be evaluated for its efficacy, efficiency and impact on society. Finally, the study results must be built into coherent recommendations for health policy, and these recommendations must be used to change the practice of health care and health care planning.

Appropriate care
(targets 26–31)

These six targets outline the design and structure of a system for the delivery of appropriate health care, based on well developed, integrated primary health care. The quality of care should be assured through the systematic assessment of technology and evaluations of health workers' performance. Appropriate care is so important in achieving health for all that it is a basic theme of the targets and a priority in research that has already been discussed in part.

Successfully redirecting a health care system primarily depends on political will and decision-making. Research on health systems can be an important source of advice for policy-makers. It can also help to ease the transition from the hospital to primary health care as the centre of health care systems. Researchers can draw policy-makers' attention to considerable amounts of existing data.

The central research questions are:

- how to develop a system of primary health care adapted to countries' central and local circumstances;

- how to allocate resources according to people's needs;

- how to achieve a proper balance of resources between primary health care and hospital and specialized care;

- how to mobilize community participation;

- how to educate health care personnel in teamwork and the management of services;

- how to make primary health care more acceptable to patients and how to use it to support lay care and self-help; and

- how to assess the quality of care and how to use the results to improve the acceptability of health services to patients and the feedback to health personnel.

22

These eight targets have two aims, as closely related as the two sides of a coin. The first is to safeguard human health from potential harm resulting from biological, chemical and physical agents, including hazardous waste. The second is to enhance the quality of life by providing people with clean water and air, safe food, and pleasant living and working conditions.

Healthy environment (targets 18–25)

Increased research is needed to:

— study specific agents and their effects

— provide information on risks and their management

— develop integrated monitoring systems

— promote community participation in work for environmental health.

More basic research is needed on health hazards in the environment, their causes and possible means of preventing them. This work should include studies on genetic variability, ecogenetics and environmental genotoxicology. The interaction of different agents has to be investigated at the level of the intact animal, the organ and the cellular and subcellular systems. Other important topics are the interaction of low-dose and long-term exposure to agents and combined exposure to various risks.

A comprehensive and internationally comparable inventory is needed of the available data on both environmental agents and their effects on the environment and health. Such an inventory should also review the data for their usefulness in preventing environmental risks and protecting health. The data collected should include facts that will help political decision-makers to manage risks and to improve regulations and laws to protect the environment.

Sometimes the best way of protecting human health may be to monitor the environment. At other times, it may be better to monitor adverse effects in the population, preferably before symptoms are recognized. Monitoring must cover all aspects of environmental health in which risk management is called for. Research must show what is to be monitored and how this should be done to ensure that the information is valuable in decision-making.

Finally, the public must be encouraged to take a greater part in presenting, discussing and handling environmental health issues. Studies based on the behavioural and social sciences must identify ways to provide people with better information on health concerns and risk factors. They must also show how to establish community participation in environmental risk management. This will result in a greater desire for safety, and decision-makers will take greater care to ensure that they consider environmental health when planning and assessing new developments.

Lifestyles conducive to health (targets 13–17)

Lifestyles (which are largely determined by the individual, societal and environmental factors that prevail in a society and the different groups composing it) strongly influence health or illness. The five targets on lifestyles recognize these facts. The social and behavioural sciences have two important roles in research on lifestyles. They should assess the effects of various lifestyles on health and promote the concept of healthy lifestyles as the normal way of life in a society.

Increased research is needed on:

— indicators of lifestyles

— lifestyles that damage health (risk behaviour)

— lifestyles that improve health (positive health behaviour)

— induced changes in lifestyle (health promotion).

Valid, reliable and sensitive indicators of health-related behaviour are needed to discover exactly how lifestyles affect health. In particular, completely new measures should be developed to assess such factors as positive health behaviour, social support and social integration, and chronic stress arising from work and from roles imposed on people according to their sex.

Intervention programmes must be based on a thorough understanding of what health-damaging behaviour does to the person who engages in it, and the purpose it serves for the individual and

24

society. Research can provide the knowledge needed. In addition, all intervention programmes should be scientifically evaluated.

The emphasis on positive health is a promising new approach to improving people's health. It implies a fundamental change of direction for health research: a shift from the study of disease and treatment to the study of health and factors that promote it. A clearer concept of positive health is urgently needed. Descriptive and analytical studies of how certain lifestyles can benefit health are equally important.

The deepest motive for studying current lifestyles is the intention to change them, to promote lifestyles that enhance health and to reduce those that damage it. Large-scale attempts to modify widespread behaviour will, however, cause ethical and practical problems. These can be solved only if new forms of community participation are developed for planning and running intervention programmes and the research projects that will accompany them.

Targets 1–12 aim at reducing health inequities, morbidity and mortality from specific causes, and at improving the quality of life.

Increased research is needed:

Fundamental requirements for health for all (targets 1–12)

— to improve the data base

— to redirect research towards public health needs

— in the forms of longitudinal studies and small area data.

Setting up a reliable data base on inequities, morbidity, mortality and the quality of life is of primary importance. It is needed to provide information for the monitoring of progress towards the targets.

Priority should be given to research projects aimed at prevention of, treatment of or rehabilitation for common diseases. Research that offers chances of improving the quality of life is equally important. Research objectives should not therefore be limited to issues affecting only selected target populations, such as hospital patients, but should extend to problems of morbidity in

25

primary care and the community. While better, broader assessments of high-powered modern technology are urgently needed, more attention should also be paid to diagnostic and therapeutic strategies and evaluative research in primary health care.

Chronic, disabling disease causes many major public health problems in the European Region, which will be augmented by the aging of the population. Research is urgently needed on the course and outcome of different forms of illness over periods of years, the relevant risk factors, and the effectiveness of different forms of intervention, even though the results of such studies may not be available by the target date.

To give a wider focus to health policy, health surveys should include people's perceptions of their health and that of their families. Both retrospective and, in most cases, prospective longitudinal studies will also be necessary. Small area data on the need for health services, and their provision and results, are required to plan and evaluate intervention programmes. These data should be collated with relevant community or regional data.

2

Support for
health development

The targets in this chapter detail the requirements for changes in the thinking and working practices of everyone whose contribution is needed to achieve health for all. The first requirement, of course, is research strategies, but they are thoroughly discussed elsewhere. The others are: a health policy committed to the principles of health for all (target 33), effective management (target 34), a reliable information base (target 35), well trained and motivated health personnel (target 36), support from professions outside the health services (target 37), and health care technology that effectively and acceptably meets people's needs (target 38).

These targets must be reached first. Their date for completion — before 1990 — confirms this fact. The support measures they call for are needed to create the necessary conditions for health development. All the research proposals in this chapter will not, however, be equally important in all countries. Depending on national and local circumstances, research should be directed towards removing the most serious obstacles and filling in the most serious gaps in knowledge. The methods that promise to yield results most rapidly should be selected, even at the expense of detail and comprehensiveness.

Time frame

27

Nevertheless, the deadline set for these targets does not mean that research not finished or perhaps not even started by 1990 should be abandoned. Many of the studies proposed will, in fact, have to be continued or followed up long after this date. The deadline actually reflects the urgency of studies that will provide the necessary basis for healthy policy and research into other fields.

Close links to other targets

The regional targets are so closely related that recommendations for research on them overlap. Much of what is recommended for the six targets in this chapter will be further discussed in other chapters. This is particularly true of Chapter 3, on appropriate care, which outlines the necessary steps for developing a health care system based on primary health care. The present chapter takes a more general view of the health care system as a whole, as a part of society. It thus gives a systematic outline of research needs, which are later developed into detailed research proposals.

How and who to act on research recommendations

Naturally, many of the research recommendations outlined in this analysis will have to be adapted to meet national priorities and local circumstances. This is particularly true for research into measures to support health development. Perhaps more than anywhere else, each Member State is on its own in this area. The research recommendations in this chapter are thus rather general. Some quite conspicuously lack the specificity required before actual research can be started. The most demanding part of designing research on support measures is left to the policy-makers and health researchers in each Member State.

A glance at the topics dealt with in this chapter shows that the main disciplines involved will be the social, behavioural, pedagogical and organizational sciences. In most Member States, however, these disciplines have not yet been drawn sufficiently into health research. The existing health research infrastructure must be changed or expanded. This will attract more contributions from disciplines without a traditional link to health research and foster wide interdisciplinary cooperation to support health for all.

28

> *Before 1990, all Member States should ensure that their health policies and strategies are in line with health for all principles and that their legislation and regulations make their implementation effective in all sectors of society.*
>
> *This could be achieved if all countries were to make a systematic review of their health policies and health legislation in the light of the regional health for all strategy and targets, and to develop health for all strategies and targets and amend or extend their health legislation accordingly, taking due account of the specific legal, political and structural conditions in each Member State.*

**Target 33.
Policies for
health for all**

The task

Many targets echo this call for Member States to make policies in line with the principles of health for all. In fact, policy is a central concern of each group of targets. Eight targets suggest that governments make policies for:

— making primary health care the hub of the health care system (target 26)

— monitoring and controlling pollution (targets 20–23)

— helping people to choose healthy lifestyles (target 13)

— developing people's health potential (target 2)

— equity in health (target 1).

Target 33 envisages four types of action: an official and explicit commitment of government to the objective of health for all; legislation that adapts the health for all strategy to national, regional and local circumstances; work to enlist the support of influential political and social organizations; and the establishment of health councils whose members represent a wide range of interests in health care and in political, economic and social affairs.

What can scientific research do to stimulate and support these policies?

It can contribute in two main areas: monitoring and evaluating the development of health policy, and showing the value of policies for health for all.

Priority topics   *Monitoring and evaluating policy development.*   In deciding on health policy, government officials and health authorities have to reconcile many different (and possibly conflicting) interests and demands in health and other sectors of society. As a result, the original intentions of the strategy for health for all may be watered down or the aims reinterpreted, to make them less challenging and more easily compatible with other, conflicting interests. Health researchers can play an important role as advocates of the original intentions and principles of the strategy. As advisers to governments or to funding organizations, scientific experts from all disciplines could use their personal and professional prestige to buttress the strategy, especially its less easily accepted parts.

More specifically, policy analyses and health systems research could influence the making of health policy. They should aim first at clearly describing health policy as outlined by the targets. In principle, at least, every government in the European Region has endorsed policies for health for all. Continuous monitoring of national health policy should be used to point out shortcomings and gaps in the implementation of such policies. Policy analyses could heighten the awareness of discrepancies between an officially proclaimed policy and its translation into action. Analyses could also define areas in which action is still needed.

The methods of process evaluation should also be applied to the making of health policy, to analyse the obstacles to changing national health policy and to seek ways of overcoming them. Successes and failures in health policy development should also be assessed. The reasons for failure, the parts played in the process by different groups and the influences of other sectors of society should be analysed. This should make the process of health policy formulation clearer to the people involved, to professionals and to the general public. An assessment of the influence of scientific research on the process of developing health policy should be

30

included in these studies. Such analyses could have useful side effects. Public awareness of health policy issues could be increased and, in turn, could help to mobilize public and professional support for policies in line with health for all.

Showing that policies work. Probably the best way to promote policy decisions in favour of a health care system guided by the principles of health for all is to prove the value of such a system. All health care systems share three overall objectives: effectiveness, cost-efficiency and equity. Policy-makers and the various interest groups involved in decision-making would be convinced of the worth of a health care system based on primary health care if they had clear proof that it is the best way to reach those objectives. Ways must be found to analyse health policies found successful in Member States and to determine the extent to which they would be useful in other countries.

Different health policies can be compared in several ways. Research can determine how close an existing health care system comes to meeting its own objectives, or compare trends in health policy development in various countries over a period of time. The third alternative is to analyse different ways of organizing a health care system. This would allow for projections of both the resources needed and the results expected, and demonstrate the consequences of decisions for different types of health policy.

All analyses must cover six main sets of variables:

- cultural, social, economic and environmental conditions known to affect health (such as minimum income, poverty and unemployment, sanitation and water supply, and air pollution);

- factors in the health system that reflect the characteristics of different health policy alternatives (such as the presence of components of primary health care, the distribution of resources between hospitals and primary health care, and the provision of support and rehabilitative services in the community);

- indicators of positive health and of patterns of mortality, morbidity and disability;

- indices of effectiveness, allowing an assessment of the degree to which services meet health care needs;

- input variables (including cost-assessment); and

- indicators of equity in the provision of services (their availability according to need, and the extent to which various groups in the population find them accessible, affordable and acceptable).

As this incomplete list clearly shows, a detailed and comprehensive comparison would take years to complete. An appropriate analytical model for evaluating alternatives for health systems must therefore be developed if the powerful tools of evaluative research are to be used in making decisions on health policy in the foreseeable future. The first and most important task for research is thus to single out major variables. These can serve as provisional or proxy indicators of a whole set of related variables. It must be possible to obtain reliable data on them without too much additional effort.

Once a set of essential variables has been established and defined in practical terms, the consequences of different health policy decisions can be identified. This could prove the worth of health policies guided by the principles of health for all. It would certainly be the greatest support research could give to such policies and to the health care system that should grow out of them.

Target 34. Planning and resource allocation

Before 1990, Member States should have managerial processes for health development geared to the attainment of health for all, actively involving communities and all sectors relevant to health and, accordingly, ensuring preferential allocation of resources to health development priorities.

Such a process should cover the systematic planning, monitoring and evaluation of health for all activities, with due regard to the specific legal, political and structural characteristics of each country.

The Member States are asked to create health policies aimed at   *The task*
establishing a health care system guided by the principles of health
for all. When they have done so, how are they to translate policy
decisions into an organizational structure that works? Target 34
answers this question.

Member States are to develop or strengthen the ways in which
they manage health development, in order to make, carry out and
evaluate strategies for health for all. Because legal and administrative structures differ among Member States, these strategies
could take the form of either a systematic health plan or a less
formal, yet coherent, set of rules, regulations and incentives. The
organizational strategy should take as its leading objectives the
principles of health for all (promoting health; reducing inequity;
increasing the effectiveness, efficiency and quality of the health
system; and strengthening community participation and intersectoral cooperation in health affairs).

An adequate organizational strategy should:

- aim at reducing health hazards and improving people's health;

- be capable of selecting long-term solutions that favour health
  promotion and the prevention of ill health;

- be amenable to cost-effectiveness analysis; and

- ensure that the people who use and provide services also take
  part in planning, implementing and evaluating them.

Such an organizational strategy gives rise to several main management tasks. First, priority objectives and targets must be defined to solve the most urgent health and health service problems in
each country. Next, the main types of activity to be undertaken in
the health sector and in other relevant sectors must be indicated,
along with the authorities to be responsible for carrying them out.
Special attention must be given to organizational measures to
develop or strengthen primary health care and to ensure its integration with hospital and specialized care. (This topic is more
fully discussed in Chapter 3.) Finally, and perhaps most important,

33

priorities in the allocation of resources must be set; effective machinery must be established for continuously monitoring and assessing resource allocation.

Member States should be encouraged to use a network of experts and institutions to ensure that management practices are effective. This network could help to: develop and apply appropriate management processes; give adequate training to all the people who will be actively involved in organizational change; involve communities in decision-making; allocate resources preferentially to local communities to develop or strengthen primary health care; and ensure the continuous evaluation of processes and results of organizational change and make further changes if necessary.

WHO is prepared to help European Member States build better management processes. The Regional Office for Europe will support individual countries, if requested, and use its network of national institutions for developmental and educational activities aimed at improving management processes. In addition, WHO will encourage countries to share information on and expert knowledge of management problems and will coordinate corresponding research at the regional level.

Priority topics   The research work needed to facilitate and support effective management will be detailed in the discussion of several other targets. The main organizational task is to establish or strengthen a fully developed primary health care sector and to integrate it with hospital and specialized care. Chapter 3, on appropriate care, contains a number of specific research proposals for various aspects of this task.

Chapter 3 outlines the structural changes needed in the health care system and the general contributions to be sought from organization, management and health services research. The contribution of research to solving specific problems in managing health systems is detailed under targets 26–31. The present chapter discusses more general recommendations.

Using expertise from other sectors in health management.   Health management should make full use of theories and practices

34

developed outside the health sector, especially those of industry and commerce. Although these sectors have different objectives, they share similar problems of managing complex organizations. In industry and commerce, successful solutions have been found to such problems as:

- how best to allocate scarce resources to attain well defined objectives;

- how to structure authority and decision-making so that people at all levels become committed to their work and use their creative potential;

- how to channel the flow of information so that essential information is readily available to management at different levels;

- how to set up programmes of basic and continuing education adapted to an organization's objectives and needs; and

- last, and perhaps most important, how to establish machinery for continuously evaluating an organization's performance and for ensuring rapid feedback to be used in management decisions.

Briefly, at present management theory has three broad principles: management by objectives, delegation and decentralization, and a systemic approach (continuous evaluation and feedback).

If the experience gained in the business world from these management problems were made available to the health care system, the complex and demanding task of restructuring the system in accordance with the principles of health for all could be solved. The cooperation of successful industrial managers would be a desirable aid to the long-term health services research groups that should be established in Member States (see Chapter 3). Management experts from outside the health sector should be included in the network of experts and institutions that Member States should use to develop and apply appropriate management processes. Care must be taken, however, to safeguard the specific character of health services research and its emphasis on people.

Studying health services and organization. Adequate health management should follow a clear strategy with well defined objectives. It should aim at getting results and should involve other sectors of society and the users of services. Finally, responsibilities and functions at different levels should be clearly defined. Detailed descriptive analyses should be made of management processes at various levels of the health care system. They could determine whether current practice meets standards for adequate management, and where improvements are most urgently needed. Such descriptive case studies might conclude, for example, that health care has no single, clearly defined objective but rather multiple goals in its different components and levels. The studies might also show that the explicit and implicit aims in health care conflict, or that the aims of certain interest groups dominate the whole system. Case studies could also point out the adverse effects of management practices, reveal where normative regulations raise obstacles to a dynamic approach, and suggest the changes necessary. It would be wise to draw extensively on the expertise of professional managers and management consultants for clear assessments of current management practices in the health system.

In addition, comparative case studies of particularly effective management processes could be useful. They could determine and describe the essential dimensions of effective management in practical terms. They could also be used to develop a standard set of incentives to the adoption of more effective management practices.

Pilot studies using tracers could test alternative models of management processes, determine where innovative impulses get bogged down in the system, and explore the impact of new incentives and regulations. These could help solve certain management problems (such as defining objectives and goals, structuring the flow of information for management, and establishing means for rapid feedback of information on performance so that organizational changes can be made). Besides providing criteria for more effective management practices, the results of such pilot studies could be used to develop and test models of health management

36

problems. These in turn would facilitate future decisions on management issues. The models could also be used in the training of administrators and health personnel for management.

The question of training various kinds of health professional for management deserves particular attention. Studies should assess the content, processes and results of existing training programmes for management at the different levels of the health care system. They should also point out essential elements for change in new developments in curricula.

Studies are also needed to analyse the effects on management of health legislation and the administrative regulations that follow. Many well intended laws and regulations lose their original impact. When introduced into administrative and management practice, they meet with unforeseen obstacles or produce unintended side effects that impede their implementation. Regulations for cost-containment may serve, in some countries at least, as an example of this type of problem. Process analyses of the implementation of selected health laws and regulations could pinpoint any obstacles and harmful side effects.

Health insurance systems and remuneration schemes are particularly important topics. Studies should assess their effect on the provision and use of services, on the preferences given to certain patterns of care, on unmet health care needs, on the attractiveness of different health professions, on equality of access to health services and, as a result, on health. Although many probably conflicting interests have to be taken into account, changes in these schemes could provide effective incentives for a widespread change in the provision and use of health services.

Intersectoral research. Establishing health services based on the principles of health for all will affect other sectors of society than health. These will include: social legislation and social services; education; health insurance; housing and town planning; environmental protection in industry and agriculture, in the home, on the roads and in vehicles; and the production and marketing of foodstuffs. It is therefore highly important that intersectoral research be promoted and researchers in other sectors mobilized to study the effects on health of their own fields of work.

**Target 35.
Health information
systems**

> **Before 1990, Member States should have health information systems capable of supporting their national strategies for health for all.**
>
> *Such information systems should provide support for the planning, monitoring and evaluation of health development and services, the assessment of national, regional and global progress towards health for all and the dissemination of relevant scientific information; and steps should be taken to make health information easily accessible to the public.*

The task

More detailed, reliable indicators are needed to achieve almost every target. Because adequate information is a prerequisite for making decisions on health policy and for evaluating the existing health care system and any structural changes in it, studies are urgently needed to determine the gaps in the information needed. Research should then concentrate on filling these gaps, to provide health policy-makers and managers with the facts they need to start health for all development. The next task for research is to build up more detailed and comprehensive information systems.

Specific research requirements for the various indicators are discussed in later chapters. A framework for pointing out the research needed to yield health information is given here.

Priority topics

Current health information systems. The processes and results of actual health information systems should be carefully evaluated at national, regional and local levels for:

- the validity of the kinds of data contained (morbidity, disability and positive health; the quality, accessibility and acceptability of services; indicators of needs for health services);
- their adequacy for monitoring health for all development;
- their reliability and accuracy;

- their usefulness for decision-making in health policy, health management, diagnosis and treatment;

- the pertinence of the data on health services;

- the flow of information within and between levels of health care (primary, hospital and specialized care); and

- the feedback of information to and its interpretation by the public.

The analyses should pick out the strengths and weaknesses of today's health information systems. They should indicate the improvements needed, such as new information and better procedures for the collection, retrieval and interpretation of data, or for the flow of information. Special attention should be given to the economics of health information. The cost-effectiveness and cost-efficiency of current information systems should be assessed.

In addition, more must be known about the information that health policy-makers and leading administrators actually use to make decisions. Descriptive studies, using interviews and participant observation, should assess the sources and content of such information. These studies could support health policies based on the principles of health for all.

Adequate information for the people is an obvious prerequisite for their participation in work for health for all. Research can contribute to improved public information by discovering how much various groups know about health. Studies should evaluate health information campaigns aimed at the general public and determine how much of the content of the popular media pertains to health. Research should also present important findings to the public for discussion.

New information needs. The wide array of new indicators needed calls for considerable research by all scientific disciplines related to health. The most important new indicators will describe: health status, health behaviour, needs for health services, the health services provided, the variation of services according to social characteristics (such as poverty, unemployment and social disadvantages), and the effectiveness and efficiency of care.

Studies are needed to determine the content of all the recommended new indicators; to test their validity and reliability; to set up procedures for the collection, retrieval and analysis of the resulting data; and to devise channels for an effective flow of information to the appropriate recipients. The general public, patients, communities, health care personnel, health researchers, managers and health policy-makers all need information if they are to play their parts in achieving health for all.

Ways of collecting data. Collecting data is expensive. Comparative studies on the advantages and disadvantages of the various methods of data collection should point out the most suitable and efficient ways of obtaining reliable information on specific indicators. For example, indicators of poverty and unemployment may call for a population-based survey or a micro-census. Indicators of health behaviour, nutritional patterns and health status could be assessed by interviews in sample surveys in communities. The same methods could be used where health care is provided, to measure client satisfaction and the quality of services.

The links between different information systems and the compatibility of data from different sources are particularly important issues. The designers of new indicators or data collection systems must take care to ensure that they are compatible with existing data and with the systems of other institutions or sectors.

The possibilities for secondary analysis of data stored by hospitals, insurance companies, and sickness funds should receive special emphasis. These data could reveal much about trends in health development, the results of treatment, the accessibility of services, health inequities, and the effects of unemployment. Once the institutions agree to cooperate and effective methods for data analysis are developed, secondary analysis can be a rapidly accessible and relatively inexpensive source of information. Such analysis must not proceed, however, until the right of patients and care providers to privacy is ensured.

40

Information for primary health care.   Since hospital information systems are well developed in most countries, research should concentrate on the needs for information in primary care. Criteria for services needed by special population groups (such as the elderly, the chronically ill, the disabled, the disadvantaged or socially vulnerable groups) must be established and the corresponding data kept up to date. Screening methods must be developed to find people whose needs are neglected.

Research projects employing the techniques of action research and participant observation are probably best for determining the information needed for primary health care. They could also find the best way of obtaining the required data. "User-friendly" computerized methods of collecting, analysing and using clinical and administrative data should be developed; they would be particularly useful in primary health care.

Cost-effective information.   A huge amount of information is needed at all levels of the health system and great resources are necessary for the development of new indicators and the collection of new data. The cost-effectiveness of gathering and using health information is thus an important issue. Criteria must be devised for weighing the advantages gained through the availability of specific data against the cost of collecting and analysing them.

Again, the possibility of secondary analysis of existing data should be carefully explored whenever the introduction of new indicators is considered. Methods should be developed to balance eventual losses of information against savings of resources in time, money and personnel.

The ethics of information.   Because of the rapid development of electronic information technology, the protection of personal data has become a highly sensitive issue, particularly in matters relating to health. Ways must be found of ensuring citizens' rights to have access to data on their own health, and to protect their privacy by having a say in decisions on the use of such data.

41

At the same time, researchers obviously need to be able to get statistical data on health for planning and evaluation. Some way of linking different sets of data on the same person must be found. This is especially important for long-term studies and those relating health to sociodemographic characteristics. This research requirement can easily conflict with people's right to the protection of personal data. This conflict often handicaps health-related research, and researchers, as well as health administrators and the public, seem to feel growing insecurity and confusion about this issue.

National and international regulations for the use of health data in scientific investigations should therefore be created. They should strike a balance between the protection of personal data and research requirements. Techniques should be developed to prevent the misuse of data storage and linkage systems.

This issue can be settled satisfactorily only if the general public and groups with a particular interest in the protection of personal data have ample opportunities to help establish such regulations.

International comparisons of health information. International comparisons are a powerful tool of investigation in many different areas of health research. By indicating, for instance, successful policy decisions in favour of a health system based on primary care, such comparisons could support the making of such policies in other countries. Comparisons could also reveal the special shortcomings of policy decisions. In addition, experience gained from new developments in one country could be used in others.

Relevant information (on such subjects as the structure of health services, population characteristics, economic and environmental conditions, health status, health behaviour, the allocation of resources, and the outcomes of the services delivered) must be comparable within and among countries. This is the most important prerequisite for comparative studies. WHO should make full use of its international connections and its network of collaborating centres to promote an internationally compatible classification and coding of information on health and health services.

Target 36.
Planning, education and
use of health personnel

> *Before 1990, in all Member States, the planning, training and use of health personnel should be in accordance with health for all policies, with emphasis on the primary health care approach.*
>
> *This can be achieved if all countries analyse their needs for the different categories of health manpower required to implement their policies of health for all, adopt suitable health manpower policies, and decide on the numbers and educational qualifications required for each category of personnel.*

The task

The planning, education and use of health care personnel in most countries depend greatly on the approach taken to health. Any discussion of health personnel should begin by examining the approach that has shaped the health care system in which they work.

In recent years, people have tended to take a technological approach to the problems of health. In hospitals, in particular, advances in genetic research, organ transplantation, health technology and clinical pharmacology are held to promise further progress in fighting disease and increasing life expectancy. This approach inevitably demands that all health care (and thus the training of health personnel) become more and more specialized and compartmentalized. In many countries the technological approach has led to a relative glut of highly specialized personnel, especially physicians, and a lack of paramedical and care personnel (such as nurses, physiotherapists, ergotherapists, home helps and social workers).

Today, health policy-makers, health professionals and the general public are increasingly concerned about the widening distance between providers and patients and the loss of patients' individuality that have resulted from too great a dependence on technology. In many countries, a new health movement favours what may be called an ecological approach to the problems of health and health care. This approach gives priority to people's capacities for preserving and strengthening their own health, for

43

creating a healthy physical and social environment, and for caring for and supporting each other.

From this point of view emerge new needs for health, including more services that promote health, and preventive, supportive and rehabilitative services in the community. Such services will cope better with the changes in patterns of morbidity and meet the new health care needs that result. Consequently, health care personnel should centre their activities on their caring, supportive and counselling functions. The ecological approach is the core of the regional strategy for health for all.

The planning and education of health personnel thus take place in a social context marked by conflicts and contradictions. On the one hand, modern clinical health care calls for highly specialized health personnel and technology-intensive methods of treatment and care. On the other, new health care needs, arising from changes in the morbidity patterns in industrial societies and from a different understanding of the patient's role, demand broadly qualified health personnel and personnel-intensive methods of care. In addition, the need for cost-containment seems to close the door on any attempt to meet people's new health care needs by increasing the total number of health personnel.

The solution to these problems, according to targets 26–31, is to shift the focus of health care systems to primary care. Of course, this will require that personnel be shifted to that sector, along with other resources. Personnel requirements in such a health care system, and research to support them, are detailed in Chapter 3.

The strategy for health for all calls for the use of the ecological approach to health, not only in primary health care, but also in the other areas of health care and other sectors of society. Equity, health promotion and the prevention of disease, citizen participation and multisectoral cooperation are objectives for the planning and education of personnel in all sectors of the health care system. Research on health personnel is an important part of this task.

Priority topics   *New needs and work for the health professions.*   Research into epidemiology and demography should determine the health care needs of the population. This will allow an estimate of the number and qualifications of various kinds of personnel required to meet health care needs. Questions to be considered include the balance between medical and paramedical personnel, the effect on health of various physician/population ratios, and health care needs that are inadequately met at present.

Pilot studies of well run primary care units could define the activities and duties of the various health professionals working there and determine the knowledge, skills and attitudes they require.

The research methods employed should include participant observation, expert panels and group discussions between primary health care teams and the people who use their services. The results of these studies could be used to make a clearer description of job profiles in primary care services. They could also be fed into educational programmes for health personnel.

Present and future education.   The goals of the academic training of health personnel may differ widely from service requirements, consumer expectations and general socioeconomic conditions. Evaluative studies should be used to determine where serious divergences occur and thus where improvements are most urgently needed. Such studies should compare the objectives, curricula and results (in knowledge, skills, attitudes and motivation) of educational programmes for the various health professions with the objectives and service requirements of new health care needs.

Many existing educational programmes will have to be adapted to the emerging requirements of new health services. Students acquire not only knowledge and skills in their professional education but also secondary socialization. In this process they imbibe specific attitudes, motivation and values for their future work. Educational programmes should therefore strive to impart attitudes, motivation and values that attract students to primary health care and enable them to work as partners with other members of the health care team and with their patients or clients. Pedagogical research could help in this task.

A major organizational problem is how to improve relations and coordination between the health and education sectors. Closer links are needed to promote intersectoral approaches and relate educational programmes to the principles of health for all. The emerging university network for health for all provides a unique opportunity in this respect and should be fully supported in all Member States.

One additional requirement must be mentioned. Health services tend to take quite different directions in clinics and hospitals than in primary care. The differences between the technological and ecological approaches could polarize them into mutually exclusive creeds, resulting in a dangerous split between the primary and other sectors of care. The education of health personnel must strike a balance between the two approaches and foster mutual understanding and esteem.

Model educational programmes should be developed to meet new health care needs and new requirements for health personnel. The models should be carefully evaluated and used to develop adequate programmes of basic and continuing education for the various health professions.

Case studies of the success or failure of past endeavours to introduce a new system of education for health professionals, oriented towards primary health care, would be extremely valuable.

<table>
<tr><td>Target 37.
Education of personnel
in other sectors</td><td>*Before 1990, in all Member States, education should provide personnel in sectors related to health with adequate information on the country's health for all policies and programmes and their practical application to their own sectors.*

This could be achieved if public policy stressed that health protection was also a key concern for sectors other than health, and if training programmes for the personnel in such sectors stressed the reasons for actively supporting health for all activities.</td></tr>
</table>

The task Health researchers can contribute to creating support for health for all among people in occupations indirectly related to health.

46

Educational programmes. Groups such as teachers, architects, economists, engineers, journalists, actors and other entertainers, and the police can make a special contribution to health for all. A wide array of programmes can be aimed at securing their support. Research could assist mainly by evaluating such programmes, and by pointing out and publicizing particularly successful campaigns or training programmes. Pedagogical research could play a key role in adapting interdisciplinary curricula on aspects of health for use in training in the various professions.

Support from the scientific community. Of course, scientists engaged in research on problems in health for all have special opportunities and responsibilities for telling other members of the scientific community about the ideas behind the movement. Scientists should use the well established infrastructure of scientific communication at national and international levels to inform other researchers of the problems in health and health care and to enlist their support for health for all. Articles on research for health for all, published in the journals of the various disciplines, or the discussion of topics arising from the movement at the meetings of scientific societies and professional associations could be powerful tools in this work.

Before 1990, all Member States should have established a formal mechanism for the systematic assessment of the appropriate use of health technologies and of their effectiveness, efficiency, safety and acceptability, as well as reflecting national health policies and economic restraints.

This could be done if governments adopted a clear policy for the systematic and comprehensive assessment of all new technical devices designed for use in the health field, to be carried out in a manner suited to the characteristics of their countries; and if an international system for the exchange of information on this subject were set up.

**Target 38.
Health technology
assessment**

47

The task   Both health professionals and the public often have conflicting attitudes towards the benefits and dangers of technological development in health care. On the one hand, the successes of modern health care doubtless lie, to a large extent, in the use of technology to fight disease. On the other hand, many feel growing concern about the dangers of the uncontrolled growth of health care technology. One obvious reason for such concern is the recent explosion in the costs of health services.

Cost-containment is not the only issue. Technology has a powerful influence on the structure and functions of society, on people's expectations and behaviour and on social relations. Health technology has undoubtedly changed the relationship between health professionals and the people who use their services. Some fear that the emphasis on technology may lead to a perception of a person as an object composed of various interrelated organ systems, for each of which a different medical specialist is competent and responsible. This would inevitably turn health personnel into highly specialized bioengineers and biotechnicians. Further, the increased sophistication of health technology obviously decreases people's ability to make informed choices and participate in decisions on their own treatment and care. In sum, people within and outside the health sector fear that the uncontrolled growth of health technology could dehumanize health care for both the providers and the users of services.

These economic and social considerations have shown the need to establish ways of systematically assessing health technology, to control its growth and avoid unwanted consequences and side effects. In the past decade, the interdisciplinary field of health technology assessment has begun to emerge, fostered by developments in the United States. It is also developing rapidly in Europe. WHO has begun and supported the building of a European network for health technology assessment.

In this discussion, the term health technology is not restricted to hardware. It is used in a broader sense, to include drugs and the medical and surgical procedures used in health care. The assessment of health technology can be defined as a process of multidisciplinary

48

research involving disciplines such as health care, engineering, economics, the social sciences and health systems research. It aims at determining the short-term and long-term effects of health technology to provide a rational basis for decisions on its introduction and use.

Consequences of health technology. Health technology has three **Priority topics** main types of consequence: health outcomes, economic consequences and social and ethical side effects.

The health outcomes of technology are its relevance, effectiveness and acceptability. Research must determine whether a particular technology meets people's health care needs, whether and how well it works, and whether it is suitable for use under existing conditions.

A variety of methods are available for assessing the effects of technology on health. They range from preclinical biochemical and animal tests to the most powerful tool, the randomized controlled trial, which can provide detailed and reliable information on the effects on health of the device, drug or procedure tested but requires considerable amounts of time, money and research personnel. Improved methods are needed mainly at an intermediate level. Clinical observation and comparative case analysis, for example, should be further developed. The solution of the problems of these methods (observational bias, placebo effects and attribution of causality) would speed up the assessment process and allow the evaluation of more minor technology. In addition, these methods could be applied more easily in ordinary clinical settings and thus improve the measurement of effectiveness.

Safety and acceptability to the client are relative concepts that refer to an implicit risk–benefit ratio. If the benefits of a certain technology are high, a relatively high risk and burden for the patient may be acceptable. As the case of chemotherapy for cancer shows, however, this ratio is often difficult to establish and assess. How many additional months of survival, to be expected with what probability, compensate for how much additional suffering and loss of quality of life? Further research is clearly needed on risk–benefit assessment.

49

In most countries, regulations and laws on the clinical use of drugs differ from those on devices and procedures. The need to introduce controls on procedures analogous to those on drug prescribing and marketing should be carefully examined in each country. Particular attention should be paid to the risks of misusing new technology (such as genetic screening) and to ways of ensuring that it is used appropriately.

The economic consequences of health technology are receiving much attention. Efficiency is a relative term. The costs of a drug, device or procedure matter less than its worth (its effects on health) in relation to the costs and worth of other methods. The assessment of effects on health is therefore a prerequisite for any assessment of efficiency. To be made comparable, health effects can be assigned a monetary value (through cost–benefit analysis), expressed in terms of a desired result (such as years of life gained, degree of disability and dependency reduced) or both.

Since assigning a monetary value to health is obviously difficult, further improvements in methods are needed. The objective measurement of the health outcomes of various kinds of health technology is particularly important. Special emphasis should be laid on such indices of outcome as people's quality of life, independence in the activities of daily living and participation in making decisions about their own care and lives.

The second set of variables to be included in an assessment of efficiency concerns the measurement of costs. Despite the progress that health economists have made, cost-assessment remains a complex task. The direct costs of health care services must be considered side by side with the indirect costs, for both the patient and society, caused by losses in wages, productivity and tax revenue. Assessing the costs of a particular procedure or a single service component is especially difficult because care tends to consist of many closely interrelated activities.

The assessment of costs in primary health care should be a field of special concern for health economics. Again, the most convincing argument in favour of a health care system based on primary care would be clear proof of its advantages. Such proof must, of course, include an assessment of costs and efficiency.

The third kind of consequence — the social and ethical side effects of health technology — can in general be described fairly easily. The growth of health technology has certainly had some unfortunate social consequences, such as too great a reliance on experts, the loss of people's autonomy in health matters and the alienation of the users of services from the providers. These consequences are, however, extremely difficult to measure. They also vary from one technology to another. For example, how much additional loss of the patient's autonomy results, say, from the introduction of nuclear magnetic resonance scanners? How is the prestige and acceptability of a health care setting affected by having or not having a scanner?

The greatest uneasiness about the development of health technology is directed towards costly high technology. This includes machinery and procedures such as lithotripters, gene technology, resuscitation, *in vitro* fertilization and artificial organ transplants. The technology used in primary health care can also have social consequences.

The whole primary care approach promises not only to help to contain costs in the long term but also, and perhaps more important, to promote equity in health, support for socially vulnerable groups, patient participation in decision-making, self-reliance, partnership and teamwork in health care, and more social integration for the elderly, the disabled and the mentally ill. An assessment of the social consequences of technology in primary care is thus a high priority. Key concepts in primary care must be clarified and given practical definitions. Methods for establishing the relationships between changes in procedures and outcome must be developed. Finally, studies are needed to compare the social consequences of primary care procedures with those of other approaches. After all, the strategy for health for all and primary health care are intended to change social structures, relations and patterns of behaviour.

The spread of health technology. Much more needs to be known about the processes of diffusion of health technology if the spread of one kind of technology is to be encouraged and the wide use of others is to be limited.

Within certain limits, laws can control the spread of technology. In many instances, however, the available evidence is not sufficient to justify legal steps, or a whole area of concern, such as the quality of life or social consequences of technology, may lie outside the law. In such instances, more informal ways of influencing the diffusion of health technology must be found. Case studies should therefore try to discover the decisive factors in the development, introduction, widespread use and abandonment of health technology. Concepts such as "technology push" and "demand pull" need further clarification, and the roles played in diffusion by health insurance systems, remuneration schemes, medical technical industry, medical leaders, the mass media and consumer expectations should be analysed.

Steps in health technology assessment. The process of assessing health technology is usually divided into four consecutive steps: selection, testing, synthesis and dissemination. All four need improvement.

Because the kinds of health technology in use or development are many and resources for technology assessment are few, methods are needed for the systematic selection of technology particularly in need of assessment and the setting of priorities for research in this field.

To contribute to the health for all strategy, technology relevant to the health care needs of the population and intended for widespread use in primary care should clearly have high priority for assessment. Comparisons of the technology used in primary care with that used in hospitals for the solution of similar problems would be particularly useful. Cost must be another criterion for selection. This does not necessarily mean that only expensive technology is chosen for assessment. The excessive use of less costly devices (such as autoanalysers) or procedures (such as the prescribing of certain drugs) may be far more expensive, for example, than all the nuclear magnetic resonance scanners put together.

In some instances, technology already in widespread use should be selected. In others, research should concentrate on assessing new technology. In yet other cases, the effects, consequences and side effects of technology still in development should be estimated.

A promising selection method would be to consider concrete situations or problem areas. For example, the European Perinatal Study Group included an assessment of perinatal technology in its study of birth in Europe.[a] Another fruitful approach would be to review the whole array of technology currently employed and to determine that most in need of assessment or most likely to be misused.

A systematic set of criteria for establishing selection priorities should be developed. A way to rank the technology selected for assessment should also be defined. International cooperation is an indispensable condition for these tasks.

Testing is the second step. For this phase, empirical measures must be established to evaluate the effectiveness, safety, efficiency and social consequences of the device, drug or procedure selected. Special attention must be paid to the problem of the indiscriminate use or misuse of technology, so that guidelines for more appropriate use can be developed. Scientific methods for assessing the safety and efficiency of drugs and, to a lesser extent, devices are relatively well developed. Improved methods are needed to assess procedures and to measure their effectiveness, efficiency, appropriateness to the situation and, above all, social consequences.

The third step in assessment is synthesis. Test results must be translated into recommendations on the further development,

---

[a] *Having a baby in Europe.* Copenhagen, WHO Regional Office for Europe, 1985 (Public Health in Europe, No. 26).

introduction (including possible limitations), and widespread use or abandonment of the technology in question. This task is especially difficult if testing yields conflicting results on the various dimensions of assessment. What recommendation should be given, for instance, in the case of two alternative procedures, if one is more efficient but has unwanted social consequences?

A synthesis of available knowledge on a particular technology can be established in a number of ways. Among them are literature reviews, expert panels, hearings, Delphi techniques, discussions in scientific journals and professional societies, and consensus-finding conferences. Each of these methods has both advantages and short-comings. An effective way of synthesizing the information derived from different scientific disciplines, to make up unequivocal policy recommendations, is still to be developed.

The information gathered in an assessment is obviously of little use if it does not reach the groups who need it. The fourth step in assessment is thus the adequate dissemination of the results of the other steps. The appropriate recipients and channels of information must be determined. Information must be presented so that the group concerned can understand it. Because some groups may be reluctant to accept the results of technology assessment, the last step in the process should include an analysis of the reasons for such reluctance and attempts to overcome it.

Infrastructure for assessment. In most European countries, the infrastructure needed for the systematic assessment of health technology is not sufficiently developed. A comprehensive assessment requires, first, more work in all relevant fields of health research, especially in health economics, health systems research and the social and behavioural sciences related to health. Further, health technology assessment (like much work for health for all) would derive direct benefit from the development of better indicators. Many research proposals made in later chapters of this book could also help to create the conditions for effective health technology assessment.

Additional efforts are needed, however. Special machinery should be established in Member States for the four steps in technology assessment. The scientific community and health authorities in Member States should actively support the emerging European network for health technology assessment. International cooperation in assessment is probably the only means of learning enough about the effects and side effects of the most important health technology.

3

Appropriate care

Although the Member States of the European Region organize their health care services in profoundly different ways, hospitals have taken the central role in health care in almost every country during the past 40–50 years. The hospital has provided leadership, controlled other levels of care and shouldered the main responsibility for the entire range of care.

The regional strategy for health for all calls for a new model for health care. Six regional targets call for a shift in the focus of health care, from the hospital to primary health care. Making this change is an enormously complex and demanding endeavour. It requires a fundamental realignment of the relationships among health service institutions and personnel.

The key element in the concept of primary health care is the provision of a broad range of integrated preventive, curative and rehabilitative services in the community. The concept particularly stresses the needs of vulnerable or underserved groups. Primary care requires cooperation and teamwork among health care personnel, individuals, families and community groups. The organizational structures needed to make this principle work will depend on local conditions in each country. Primary care means more, however, than just having a general practitioner and a referral hospital within the reach of every community.

57

The widespread establishment of comprehensive primary health care services could solve serious problems in health and health services.

First, hospital-based systems are designed to provide curative treatment for acute disease. Their very success has contributed to a change in health needs. New patterns of morbidity, the increase in chronic disorders and the aging of the population call for different health care and support services. The growing numbers of people who are elderly, mentally disturbed, chronically ill or disabled need local health and support services that will help them lead relatively normal, socially integrated lives for as long as possible. Primary health care can meet this need.

Further, the present economic climate is chilly. Resource allocation in present, hospital-centred systems produces a relatively meagre return in the shape of a general improvement in health. One of the major aims of the six targets on appropriate care is to improve that return in the future. Primary health care can strengthen preventive measures and mobilize community participation and mutual aid to support the chronically ill. A well developed primary care sector would use this ability to allocate health care resources and contain costs more effectively in the future.

In addition, closer cooperation is needed between health professionals and the people who give informal care. Primary health care would recognize and support the health care given to patients in their homes. Unpaid health workers, usually the mothers or daughters of the patients concerned, are estimated to provide up to 80% of overall health care. Clearly, informal health care deserves more attention in both health policy and research.

Finally, primary health care could lead to the discovery of new ways of ensuring community involvement in the organization and delivery of health and support services. These would help people to accept and act on the principles of self-reliance, personal responsibility and lay participation in health matters that underlie the idea of positive health and the new health movement.

Primary health care plainly offers exciting opportunities for improving health. Targets 26–31, to be completed by 1990, outline the structure of a system of appropriate health care. They begin with the principle that health care delivery should be based on primary health care services (target 26) distributed according to need (target 27). Next are specific parts of the system: the actual content of care (target 28), teamwork among the providers (target 29), and the coordination of services in the community (target 30). The final element is ensuring the quality of care (target 31). These targets make up one of the three groups of changes necessary to build health for all.

Countries that have begun to develop a primary health care sector can naturally make a smoother transition to a fully fledged new system of health care than those in which primary care has not yet been publicly discussed. Nevertheless, major structural changes will be necessary in almost every Member State. They will make special demands on health policy-making, health insurance systems, the training and career patterns of health professionals and, last but not least, public acceptance of and participation in the new system.

Changing the structure of health care

Targets 26–31 and the research recommended to attain them share a focus on the structure of the health care system. Structural changes in the health care system, however, form only the basis for the delivery of appropriate care. Whether people's health needs are fully met will, in the last analysis, depend less on the structure of the system than on how people bring it to life. Ultimate success or failure will depend on the dynamics of the health care system and, above all, on motivation and teamwork among the care providers. Close cooperation between the health care teams and the community is also important.

These decisive human factors are obviously beyond the reach of either health policy or health research planning. The discussion of research needs is therefore limited to the structure of the intended transformation, even though structure is not the only issue, and probably not even the most important.

In view of all these considerations, research has a rather delicate role to play. On the one hand, primary health care undoubtedly offers a vision that deserves full and unambiguous support from the scientific community. On the other, this does not mean the abandonment of the basic scientific attitude of critical questioning and methodical scepticism, with its demand for solid evidence. Consequently, the first and probably most important task for research would be to evaluate whether (and under what conditions) the new health care system can actually keep its promises. Research could provide an impartial analysis of successes and failures alike. This could contribute substantially to further refinement of the concept and to improvements in its use.

The task for health services research

The task is complex and time is short. How can research help stimulate and ease the transformation of health care systems?

All six targets are to be reached by 1990. The basic knowledge, concepts and principles for promoting appropriate care have been well developed since the Member States adopted them in the Declaration of Alma-Ata.[a] The issue is the implementation, not the formation, of policy and thus mainly a matter of political will, management and resource allocation. The main problem is not how to find basic knowledge but how to use it. Certain types of research can facilitate the transition or analyse the impact and value of the required reshaping of the system.

When changing an organization is the goal of a policy, the changes should be based on the theory that provides the greatest understanding of the conditions, constraints and consequences of development in an organization. This understanding can be found in organization theory, a well established applied social science. Drawing on social science disciplines (including political science, economics, psychology and sociology), organization theory is an important part of the curricula of many graduate schools of public health.

---

[a] *Alma-Ata 1978: primary health care.* Report of the International Conference on Primary Health Care. Geneva, World Health Organization, 1978 ("Health for All" Series, No. 1).

60

Research based on organization theory and its application to large organizations, including health services, differs in nature and methods from research in the natural and biomedical sciences. In organization science, research is based largely on systematic observation, comparative analyses, experience and case studies rather than on complex experimental designs or large controlled trials. These differences in method reflect a fundamental difference in the make-up of natural and social systems. People, not the laws of nature, construct social systems. Moreover, research itself can directly change the social system or subsystem under study.

Some argue that applied social sciences, such as organization and management research, are not scientific enough to provide a firm basis for action. This opinion is most often voiced against plans to use such research to study organizations or policies for the provision of public goods such as health care. In contrast, the private sector in many Member States makes full use of applied social science to achieve its management goals. Its success stories are based on precisely the "soft methodology" that policy-makers and organizations in the public sector often disdain.

This conflict over acceptability may reflect two different types of values or management goals: financial profit versus public service. It may also reflect the inherent difficulty in establishing a yardstick of organizational effectiveness in public services that can be used as readily as profit in the private sector. The growing importance of efficiency in decision-making for health, however, may very well lead to a greater appreciation of organization and management science.

Four types of research objective should be pursued: the development of a standard way to gather information, the solution of some problems of organizational development, the improvement of methods of involving different disciplines and the community in research, and the extension of health services research.

General recommendations for research

Consistent and readily usable data are lacking for several of the targets on appropriate care. Further, the information necessary for

A standard way to gather information

indicators of progress is either incomplete or unavailable. In some important cases, the available information is not relevant to the required indicators or has been compiled in a way that limits its usefulness.

This gap in clearly defined and reliable information on the development of a country's primary health care sector has rather serious consequences. Without such information, even a description of the present health service system, noting the existence or absence of components of primary care, becomes difficult. It is then impossible to assess clearly the extent to which an existing health care system is based on primary care, where improvements are most urgently needed, and the degree of progress being made.

A set of standard methods of collecting information on health services in the Region should be established. For each type of information, there should be a precise definition of what is being counted and a specific protocol for how the counting should be done. These should be made for all the types of health-related data that are either unavailable or not gathered uniformly among Member States. An important part of this task will be to provide clear, practical definitions of many of the basic concepts in health care, such as community, community representative, participation, quality of care and health care needs. At the moment these are only vaguely defined. Special care should be taken with information open to different interpretations according to people's political views or sociocultural background.

Standardized information might well have an additional advantage for health policy formulation in the Member States. The very process of assembling the data needed and restructuring national information-gathering procedures to obtain it could stimulate broad internal debate about national health policy and progress towards the regional targets.

The design and use of better information systems could follow several different courses. For example, experts from Member States could meet to ensure that the standard definitions and collection procedures developed can be implemented in national health information systems.

Realigning a health care system poses a series of major problems in organizational development. Work to solve them could benefit substantially from well designed research projects on the theory and behaviour of organizations. Projects applying the general principles of this discipline to the institutions and goals of health care systems could be particularly useful.

Research into organizational behaviour would be valuable at three levels. Studies of the health sector as a whole could help to reshape the relationship between the hospital and primary health care. Studies of primary health care could help to develop better techniques for the integration and management of the wide variety of activities in primary care. Finally, studies of local communities could help to coordinate community-based primary health care services with the activities of other sectors with an influence on health (such as social services, education and housing).

Further, applied studies of organizational behaviour at all three levels should explore two problems whose solution is vital for attaining targets 26–31. The first is how to rebuild existing health care delivery systems on the foundation of primary care. The primacy of the hospital naturally complicates this task. There has been little concrete experience in establishing and managing the new organization and structures required for a system based on primary care. Carefully designed research projects (particularly analytical case studies and comparisons between countries that can be carried out in a relatively short time) can contribute much to the speed and effectiveness of the transformation.

The second key problem is how to ensure the broadest possible consumer satisfaction with the emerging health care systems. At present, many people prefer to receive clinical treatment in a hospital rather than from primary health care personnel. The variety of explanations for this preference includes the prestige that both health personnel and patients attach to hospital specialists. One of the main tasks of organization research will be to analyse carefully the obstacles that hinder both professional and lay acceptance of primary care services, and to determine ways of

Studying the development of organizations

63

overcoming them. Further, in the face of patients' passive accept-ance of medical omniscience, new methods and procedures should be devised to encourage people to make their own independent and informed judgements on the quality of the care they receive and the efficiency of its delivery.

Making room for other disciplines and the community

Community participation and consumer satisfaction can be con-sidered not only as topics for health services research but also as features of research that should be reflected in the methods em-ployed. Research should provide ample opportunities for the people affected by the studies to take part in defining their aims, conducting the investigations and using the results. Such methods are most appropriate to social research and to the emphasis on community participation throughout the primary care approach. Methods that allow participation in research on both lifestyles and health services are not yet sufficiently developed and need to be improved.

Methods of interdisciplinary research also need development and improvement. Teamwork and the integration of services cannot be recommended or studied if, say, the allied health professions (such as nursing, physiotherapy, ergotherapy, nu-tritional therapy, health education and counselling) are excluded from the research process. The required improvements for methods of interdisciplinary research are more fully discussed in Chapter 5.

More research on health services

Most research on health services does not yet cover certain topics needed to support the establishment of an appropriate health care system. Research is still mainly construed as biomedical and, partly as a result of this, health services research seems relatively neglected. Further, a large slice of the available funds has already been given to projects in progress, so a change in the division of resources will take some time.

Under these circumstances, health services research will most probably have to be deliberately extended and supported. In many countries, the number of scientists qualified in health services research will have to be augmented. Perhaps the network of WHO collaborating centres could help to stimulate postgraduate training in health services research and to develop training courses stressing the organizational problems of the regional strategy for health for all.

Within Member States, long-term research groups should be set up to complete four important tasks. First, these research groups should develop models of a health care system based on primary health care and adapted to national and local circumstances. Detailed knowledge of examples of such systems in other countries will be needed.

Second, the groups should evaluate the processes and results of model projects. Particular attention should be given to the dynamics of structural change. How does it affect motivation and relations within the health care team and between the health care team and the community?

The third task is to analyse the existing health care system for the extent to which it is based on primary health care.

Fourth, long-term research groups should determine whether an existing health care system meets its own stated objectives. Even if shifting the focus of a national system is impossible, such an evaluation could point out important areas for improvement. Some component of primary health care might very well provide a solution. In addition, the continuous monitoring of developments in the structure of a health care system could help to determine whether any transformations were taking place. It could discover the main obstacles to further progress and how attempted changes had succeeded or failed. Finally, it could put forward alternatives to avoid future failures.

The structure of health care systems is hardly likely to change without an adequate extension of health services research. The creation of an adequate research infrastructure is a criterion for judging national political will to strengthen primary health care in the existing health care system.

**Target 26.
A health care system
based on
primary health care**

> *By 1990, all Member States, through effective community representation, should have developed health care systems that are based on primary health care and supported by secondary and tertiary care as outlined at the Alma-Ata Conference.*
>
> *This could be achieved by clear statements from the highest national authorities and political leaders of all levels of authority in the health field, backed by effective legislation, regulations and plans, making primary health care the hub of the health care system, with secondary and tertiary levels in a supporting role and only carrying out those diagnostic and therapeutic functions that are too specialized to be carried out at the primary health care level; the establishment of effective ways and means of bringing consumer needs and interests to bear on the planning and delivery of primary health care; and free discussion with all groups of health personnel, supported by appropriate modifications of health manpower policies and programmes, to obtain their full commitment and support for carrying out this policy in their daily work. Such developments should take due account of the constitutional provisions of each Member State.*

The task   The first two targets in this chapter set out the overall objectives and build the skeleton of the appropriate organization of health care systems. With target 27, target 26 outlines a programme for the development of a fully integrated health service system, spearheaded by a well organized and prestigious primary health care sector, well grounded in the local community it serves and backed by hospital and specialized care.

Target 26 is concerned with four main requirements that would guide the change in the health care system. First, political leaders and health authorities must endorse the new system. Second, health professionals and the general public must accept and respect primary health care. Third, the community must participate in planning and decision-making for health. The fourth need is appropriate policies on health personnel. Research can contribute to progress in meeting all of these.

Decisions for primary health care.   The decision to change a health care system is primarily a question of the will of political leaders and influential health authorities. Nevertheless, research could encourage such policy decisions.

Policy studies should analyse and monitor the processes of decision-making in running health systems. Are clear statements in favour of primary health care being made at all? Are any such statements followed by political and legal action? Who has the power, in theory and practice, to make decisions on specific issues? What are the priorities and interests of the most powerful institutions in strengthening primary health care? Are there conflicts of interest between and within these institutions? Could alternative models of a health system based on primary care resolve them? If the results of such analyses were published and opened to discussion by politicians, scientists and the public, a more rational approach could be taken to decision-making in health systems.

A clear descriptive analysis of an existing health care system for the presence or absence of components of primary care could encourage political and health service authorities to make necessary improvements, and could promote their willingness to make changes.

In addition, the existing health care system should be compared with successful models of primary health care. Again, a clear demonstration of the greater effectiveness and efficiency of a well developed primary care sector will substantially strengthen the political will to foster change.

Acceptance of and respect for primary health care.   Primary health care personnel and services seem to have less prestige than those in

67

hospitals or specialized care. This must change if primary health care is to take root.

Research can have relatively little direct influence on the perception of primary care among health professionals and the public. Contributions from the social sciences, however, can provide detailed knowledge of what various groups and professions feel and think about different components of primary care. Research can then determine the reasons for these views and provide a basis for strategies to strengthen the position of primary care.

Sociological and sociopsychological studies should describe in detail the perceptions, attitudes and patterns of behaviour related to primary health care among different groups of people. These groups include:

- health professionals giving primary, hospital or specialized care;

- undergraduate and graduate students in the health professions;

- the various groups of people receiving primary care services;

- family members and other unpaid health workers caring for people at home;

- the general public (specified according to such factors as age, sex, social status, educational background and involvement in other community activities); and

- the mass media and other agents of public opinion.

These descriptions should be combined with a systematic attempt to point out the main factors that account for the variations in perceptions of and attitudes towards primary health care services. In addition, the likelihood that special incentives might increase the acceptance of primary care could be assessed.

Community participation. Community participation in health services means the establishment of effective ways to bring the needs and interests of consumers to bear on the plannning and delivery of primary health care. A number of Member States have one or more forms of community representation. Some are more effective than others in influencing decisions on primary care. In general, the proportion of people interested and involved remains small, and sometimes there is little evidence of their direct participation. Research could help to establish the requirements, advantages and disadvantages of different models of community participation. Studies should also consider the possibility that specific types of local advisory panel may be taken over by the very groups or organizations they were designed to control.

Comparative organizational studies on different models of community participation or representation could provide answers to many important questions.

- What forms of representation most effectively ensure that the community's ideas have due weight in administrative decisions?

- Are alternative models being used in the European Region? Should others be designed?

- What criteria can be used to assess the value of the local council as a forum for community participation?

- Will these councils provide real local direction or will they become mere window-dressing?

- Can some models of community participation escape take-over by interest groups?

- Under what conditions are existing legal opportunities for community participation actually taken or neglected? What are the informal obstacles to formal possibilities?

- Why does the participation of certain groups (pregnant women, people with coronary heart disease and other self-help groups) work relatively well?

Policies on health personnel. Two other targets in this chapter (targets 27 and 29) deal with policies on health personnel. Their education was discussed in Chapter 2.

**Target 27.
Rational and
preferential distribution
of resources**

By 1990, in all Member States, the infrastructures of the delivery systems should be organized so that resources are distributed according to need, and that services ensure physical and economic accessibility and cultural acceptability to the population.

This could be achieved by a combination of planned development and a wide range of carefully designed incentives to direct the necessary health care resources to the primary health care services, in order to ensure that the distribution of the services and the care they provide correspond to the needs of the population; and by similarly gradually readjusting hospital resources, wherever necessary, to form a system whereby secondary and tertiary care resources are distributed in a regionalized system according to needs.

The task

This target describes the backbone of the restructuring of the health care system: the reallocation of money and people. Health care resources should be allocated according to the needs of the population, hospitals should be more rationally organized, and both financial and personnel resources should be gradually shifted from the hospital to primary health care.

These needs call for a variety of research projects in organization research and health economics.

Priority topics

Better information. The indicators proposed for this target are rather crude types of basic data on the resources used in health

70

care: expenditure; ratios between physical resources, personnel and population; the proportion of key health personnel working in primary health care; and the extent of insurance coverage. In most countries, data are not yet available (even on these simple measures) that would allow a breakdown of resource allocation for the primary care and hospital sectors. The implementation and evaluation of both regional and national health care policies require the development of standard definitions and procedures for the collection of reliable information, taking into account the proposed regional indicators.

A second priority reflects the roughness of several of the proposed indicators. There are neither indicators on needs or service outputs nor any ways to measure the relations between needs, inputs, processes and outputs, to say nothing of the much more complicated indicators of ultimate outcome. Research on and the development of unified concepts, definitions and procedures to make good these deficiencies are sorely needed. Better information is also needed on principles and notions that are sometimes difficult to measure but no less important: community representation, the distribution of resources according to need, physical and economic accessibility, and cultural acceptability.

The indicators available at present are heavily biased towards the providers of services. They fall conspicuously short in reflecting consumers' needs and interests. Research and development must strive to strike a better balance between the two in the future.

New ways to allocate resources.   Shifting resources from the hospital to primary health care is an enormous task. Three major problems require special efforts in research.

The first problem is the transfer of resources in health care. The Regional Committee's suggested solutions for target 27 include a hard policy decision giving clear preference in the allocation of resources to primary health care. This would, of course, cut down the sums assigned to the hospital sector. As the experience of several countries suggests, shifting resources remains difficult, even after such a policy is adopted.

A detailed evaluation of cases in which funds for hospitals have been transferred to primary health care (in Belgium, Finland and Sweden, for example) could provide important information on many questions. For example, what factors might increase hospitals' willingness to surrender resources? What types of incentive could be offered to hospitals and departments to improve their compliance in the change? Could certain market-style incentives be used in regional public health care systems to heighten efficiency without impairing effectiveness or equity? How might different models of a mixture of public and private financing for health services affect the reallocation of resources?

The second problem is the rationalization of the hospital sector. In the new health care systems, hospitals and specialized care are to have supporting roles. Further, hospitals should be more rationally organized. Units should have clearly defined roles and serve well defined populations. These goals will be difficult to accomplish, particularly in Member States with hospitals in which admissions are not tied to geographical or referral requirements. The process is further complicated by the deliberate pace recommended for the changes. They should be gradual, so that the local problems that may arise, particularly in employment, may be tackled.

A number of carefully designed studies, preferably covering several countries, could be undertaken within a relatively short time. These should include analyses of alternative models for organizing hospitals on a regional basis, the preconditions for their success, appropriate stages for their implementation, sources of revenue, and ways of paying physicians. Questions whose answers will seriously influence the effectiveness, financial efficiency and social equity of particular regional models should receive the greatest emphasis. Such questions include alternative methods of creating an acceptable balance between centralized authority (and hence imposed equity) and decentralized authority (and local autonomy). A second subject for research should be the organizational implications of reducing institutions. Special attention should be paid to planning, budgeting and management mechanisms for ensuring balanced reductions and the suitable transfer or retraining of personnel.

How to allocate resources according to need — the third problem — raises several questions for research into organizational behaviour. What is need-based resource planning and how should it be done? Who defines needs and what criteria are used? What roles do health care professionals, health service planners, politicians, insurance companies and consumers play in this process? Although some steps have been taken to develop need-based models, much more work is required. Further, what types of incentive or other means exist for bringing about a better demographic distribution of health personnel? Physicians and nurses in some Member States tend to be unevenly distributed. Too few work in rural and poor urban areas. Since some countries have managed to overcome physicians' resistance to less desirable postings, analytical studies should be made of successful approaches and the reasons why they have worked.

The main problem for research into organizational behaviour in primary health care is how to meet the increased requirements for staff in this sector. Many Member States will require substantial numbers of new personnel to fulfil the greater responsibilities of primary care. More nutritionists, dentists and other kinds of health and social personnel, such as physiotherapists, social workers or home helpers trained to work in the primary sector, are particularly needed. Even though many Member States have limited health budgets, they must build up adequate primary care services before they reduce services in the hospital sector. These facts give rise to a number of important issues in research on recruiting and managing primary health care personnel. For instance, estimates must be made of the personnel requirements for primary care and they must allow for the gradual expansion of services. In addition, the appropriate balance between paid and voluntary community-based care must be carefully studied. Comparative analyses of the organization and management of primary health care centres are a related task. These should ascertain the internal arrangements that ensure the most effective and the most acceptable forms of primary care.

<table>
<tr>
<td>Target 28.
Content of
primary health care</td>
<td>By 1990, the primary health care system of all Member States should provide a wide range of health-promotive, curative, rehabilitative and supportive services to meet the basic health needs of the population and give special attention to high-risk, vulnerable and underserved individuals and groups.

This could be achieved by establishing clear policies in all Member States with a description of the full range of services that the primary health care system should provide, based on the principle that most preventive, diagnostic, therapeutic and care services and activities could be provided outside hospitals and other institutional settings; modifying basic and continuing education programmes for health personnel to ensure their active support for this development; and reviewing planning, referral and incentive systems to ensure that they support these policies.</td>
</tr>
</table>

The task Target 28 puts flesh on the skeleton built in the two preceding targets. The main need is to determine the nature of a fully developed primary health care sector, the services it should offer and how to integrate services both within primary care and with hospital and specialized care. If a health service policy calls for moving away from institutions as sites for health care, for example, special attention must be paid to the additional burdens this places on family members and other unpaid health workers. Research should help to establish the content of primary health care.

Priority topics *Improving indicators.* For both designing an enlarged primary care system and assessing progress towards achieving target 28,

74

two basic types of indicator are needed. At the moment, both are unsatisfactory.

First, existing indicators of need should be assessed and new ones developed for the main target groups. This will allow estimates of the extent and nature of the services required.

Second, indicators of services offered must be improved. For example, the regional indicator on child care (the proportion of children under 5 years for whom permanent child care services are available in the community) looks deceptively simple. Nevertheless, it presents problems of definition and data collection. Additional indicators of services offered to the main target groups of primary care are needed for the planning and detailed evaluation of services.

Sinews of primary health care.   Primary health care should meet people's basic health needs in the community and give special attention to high-risk, vulnerable and underserved individuals and groups. Reaching these goals involves three main tasks that suggest a whole array of services that could be offered by a fully developed primary care sector.

First, primary health care could provide most preventive and many diagnostic, therapeutic and support services as well as (or even better than) highly specialized and expensive hospitals. Such services should therefore be transferred to primary care. They include minor surgery, immunization, physiotherapy, perinatal care, screening and laboratory tests, and surveillance of long-term treatment for the physically or mentally ill.

Second, a system of primary care is ideally suited to provide nursing and support services for elderly, chronically ill or disabled people in their homes or communities. The adverse effects of long stays in hospital could be avoided and independence, self-reliance and social integration encouraged. In addition, hospitals could be relieved of the care of long-term patients. Nursing and support services would include a variety of services such as:

● the provision of child care services and day centres or apartments for the handicapped;

75

- home help;

- nursing and outreach services for the elderly, single parents, the physically or emotionally handicapped, drug abusers and the mentally ill; and

- rehabilitation for people recovering from severe diseases (such as myocardial infarction or cancer) or treatment (such as major surgery) or living with progressive diseases (such as rheumatic diseases or multiple sclerosis).

Third, primary health care offers the chance to provide a variety of easily accessible counselling services (previously given only at scattered locations if at all). Counselling could cover health education, partnership problems, family planning, contraception and sexual problems, genetic counselling, group psychotherapy, occupational health services (for small enterprises, self-employed people and agricultural workers) and assistance for migrant workers and members of ethnic or religious minorities with problems of social integration.

Adapting primary health care to country and local circumstances. This long but not exhaustive list of desirable elements in fully developed primary health care offers Member States options from which they can choose the components that meet their needs and fit their health policies. Such choices require substantial support from health services research. The content of primary care should naturally be based on people's needs for health care. The first task is thus to determine exactly what these health needs are. This rather complex job should be tackled from several angles.

First, a practical definition of basic health care needs must be developed. It must distinguish clearly between needs and demands and between perceived needs and induced needs, aiming at an objective assessment. This framework for assessment should be particularly sensitive to the needs of vulnerable or underserved groups. Studies in epidemiology and the social sciences could then go on to estimate the extent and distribution of the health care needs of various groups in the population.

The second task is to determine which needs should be served by the different sectors of the health care system. Practical criteria must be set to point out the health care needs that primary health care can and should meet. Third, the criteria should be used to assess existing health care systems to determine what services should be shifted from the hospital to primary care or newly established in an enlarged primary care sector.

Integrating primary health care services.   Member States are faced with the problem of designing a health care system based on primary care. Broad theoretical studies could be valuable in showing how services might be organized and integrated. Such studies should draw on the principles of organization theory and examples of their application in the private sector. Integrated primary health care systems in various countries should be carefully analysed to ensure that current knowledge and experience within the Region are available to all.

This work should make it easier to answer a number of specific questions about the design of health care systems. What types of organization or administration are most effective in integrating promotive, curative, rehabilitative and support services? How can services be integrated without jeopardizing the special needs of groups requiring particular attention?

Further, how can the transition from specialized programmes to integrated and comprehensive primary health care be made or eased? This issue is very important for organizational design and for the training and use of personnel. Some services have originated separately and tend to function in isolation. Research should seek ways to integrate them with other components of primary health care.

The care of the elderly, dental health and environmental health, and services given in schools and workplaces require either particular skills or locations for delivery. How can these kinds of services be integrated? Useful comparative analyses and case studies of such services could be made fairly quickly and easily.

Primary health care services are so varied and complex that structures and processes of managing them should be investigated. Studies should determine the results of various ways of providing leadership, making decisions and allocating responsibility for health care. Ways of assigning authority and the mixture between public and private responsibilities in the organization of a primary health care system could also be compared. Should authority be split between local and country organizations? To what extent should central authority dictate policy and budget decisions to local administrative units? Should such central authority use legislation, standards or strict directives to dictate policy? Should the delivery of primary care services be completely under public direction and control? Will a form of mixed public and private control, such as contracts with private group practices, satisfy patients' demands more efficiently? What can be learned from existing contractual procedures in some Member States?

Assessing resource requirements. Studies will be needed to determine the resources that the various models of primary health care systems will probably require. Advances in care and treatment and the resulting improvement in health may make the provision of new buildings superfluous. Planners should keep this consideration in mind when deciding on the capital investment needed. Research could also inquire into possible new ways of organizing primary care services to reduce the need for training new personnel or to make use of existing personnel after retraining, particularly people now working in hospitals. Studies could also be made of different ways to provide primary care.

Interdisciplinary work by health service researchers, health economists and epidemiologists will be needed to assess the present and future resource requirements of various ways of organizing primary health care.

78

> *By 1990, in all Member States, primary health care systems should be based on cooperation and teamwork between health care personnel, individuals, families and community groups.*
>
> *This could be achieved by policies in the countries that clearly define the role that different categories of health and social personnel should play in health care; basic, specialist and continuing education programmes for health personnel that provide insight, motivation and skill in interprofessional teamwork and in cooperation with individual families, groups and communities; and health education programmes that provide a realistic picture of what services can be expected from health professionals and give help in developing lay care skills.*

The task

Although a system of appropriate care needs a sound structure, only the people who provide the care can give it life. Target 29 focuses on the providers of primary care and on the cooperation required between the providers of services, the users of services and groups in the community. An appropriate education for health professionals can contribute most to developing the motivation and skills of the primary health care team and to the team's cooperation with its clients. The team will include the whole range of professional staff that provide primary health care, including physicians, nurses, social workers, nutritionists, physiotherapists and counselling personnel. Research in four areas can help to achieve this target.

Priority topics

Indicators. Once again, the lack of informative indicators is particularly conspicuous. The sole regional indicator for this target seeks to discover whether mechanisms for ensuring the full use of human resources in primary care exist. Obviously this indicator must be translated into practical terms.

Educating health personnel for teamwork and management. In some Member States, primary care relies largely on physicians. If the full potential of primary health care is to be realized, however, all health personnel must adopt a team concept. This is a particularly sensitive issue for physicians, who have been reluctant to cooperate fully with other health care personnel. Research on organizational behaviour could help solve this problem by examining the design of educational programmes and a system of incentives that will encourage physicians and other personnel in primary health care to work as a team.

Different systems of undergraduate, graduate and continuing education for health professionals should be compared. How do these systems affect students' perception of primary health care and their motivation and ability to work with people in other health professions? In addition, case studies of failures and successes in introducing new systems of medical education specially oriented towards primary health care would be extremely valuable. Such efforts have been made in medical schools in Maastricht, Netherlands and Kuopio, Finland and in the Biomedical Science Institute in Oporto, Portugal.

The comprehensive, integrated primary health care system envisaged in the regional strategy for health for all involves different disciplines and sectors of society in providing services at different sites. For this reason, designing suitable programmes for teaching the necessary management skills to members of the primary care team is particularly important. Primary health care has been marketed as a cost-efficient alternative to hospital-based, high-technology medicine. To live up to this description, primary care personnel must drastically improve their management skills. This raises a number of issues. Research into organizational behaviour, for example, will be needed to determine what types of management education and training are best adapted to the nature of primary care. Studies should be conducted to determine whether existing management training schemes can be adapted for use in health care.

Providing acceptable services. Successful cooperation between the primary health care team and the community it serves depends on the acceptability of the services offered. Designing and running a primary care system is a waste of time if the people served do not like it and will not use it. Community participation is a two-way street. The community and the professionals must both speak and listen.

Research could help to make services more acceptable to the people who use them by assessing their needs for health care. For instance, local populations could be surveyed to discover the services they wish to see emphasized in their primary care centres. Determining whether people are satisfied with primary health care and devising procedures for trying to resolve any dissatisfaction would also be helpful. Special attention should be given to encouraging health care personnel to recognize and understand the social and family problems of the people they serve. In addition, sociopsychological studies should be encouraged. They should aim at analysing in detail the processes of interaction between providers of primary care and the users of services. Important factors in these processes include the proportion of speaking and listening on both sides, language barriers and the influence of differences in social class.

Working with lay care and self-help groups. The growth of lay care, mutual-aid and self-help groups is of special importance for the cooperation between providers of primary health care and the local community. Organization research should analyse the best ways of coordinating primary care services with the activities of such groups. An evaluation of the groups' effectiveness in prevention, health promotion, coping with illness, and providing care and support services could help to single out the tasks that the health care team should encourage them to undertake. It should also provide health personnel with valuable hints on cooperation, the acceptability of services, and people's psychosocial needs.

81

**Target 30.
Coordinating
community resources
for primary health care**

> *By 1990, all Member States should have mechanisms by which the services provided by all sectors relating to health are coordinated at the community level in a primary health care system.*
>
> *This could be achieved by recognizing the responsibility of the primary health care sector to determine what matters require special attention, change and reorientation, and to coordinate efforts in those directions; and establishing a permanent structure, e.g. a health council, in each local community, where representatives of the community itself, and health and other sectors can make joint analyses of local health plans and determine what contributions each sector should make to improving the health of the community. Such mechanisms should, of course, be developed with due regard to the various constitutional provisions of each Member State.*

The task Building a permanent structure for determining the responsibilities of each sector in improving health is mainly a question of political will and decision-making at country and, even more important, local level. Organization research can, however, play a supporting and monitoring role.

Priority topics *What is community involvement?* Definitions of the terms "local community" and "representatives of the community" are essential. The Declaration of Alma-Ata stresses the need to involve not just local officials but, above all, the local population in making decisions about primary health care. Forms of community participation range from bodies in which the community has the bare right to be heard to those in which local people have full voting rights in decision-making. Precisely defining such a politically sensitive term as community involvement may be impossible. Nevertheless, some procedures or guidelines for community participation (and appropriate mechanisms for assessing it) should be set up. These guidelines should specify what groups in the community and of care providers should be represented. In addition, research is needed to point out criteria for and indicators of community participation. These would allow the existing situation to be clearly described. The changes taking place over time could also be assessed.

Multisectoral cooperation at local level. A variety of administrative models could be adopted to carry out the multisectoral responsibilities of primary health care. They range from coordinating the individual agencies (for such services as education, social welfare and health care) to consolidating them in one local office. This structural issue is particularly relevant for social welfare services. Perhaps the most important health-related sector, these services are currently administered separately from health in most Member States. Research on organization behaviour is essential to the analysis and comparison of potential models of integration for all sorts of health-related services. These models could then be offered to Member States for consideration.

A further question is the responsiveness of primary health care to the users of the system. Intersectoral coordination should be designed to encourage people to participate, not to be passive. A more efficient local health structure dominated by care providers' concerns for job security and preserving institutions would bring little advantage to the community. Again, researchers must look for ways to ensure that the primary health care system resulting from multisectoral coordination keeps its focus on the needs of the users of services. Different kinds of community participation should be evaluated. This should make the possible alternatives more widely known and ensure that the concept is better understood.

A special problem is how to encourage occupational and leisure groups, schools, religious communities, and formal and informal associations of members of ethnic minorities to support the primary health care system. Action research programmes could determine how to do this and single out the most suitable forms of cooperation.

Advisory health councils. Target 30 proposes that advisory health councils be established as the key to coordinating health resources at local level, and to supervise the coordination of different sectors' contributions. In particular, such councils should establish priorities for the agencies that provide resources. Here, comparative organization research is needed to determine the most suitable types of organizational structure and the most effective methods of establishing them.

Target 31. Ensuring the quality of services

> *By 1990, all Member States should have built effective mechanisms for ensuring quality of patient care within their health care systems.*
>
> *This could be achieved by establishing methods and procedures for systematically monitoring the quality of care given to patients and making assessment and regulation a permanent component of health professionals' regular activities; and providing all health personnel with training in quality assurance.*

The task

The quality of care is probably the most crucial single factor in the trust put by health professionals and the public in the health care system. Hence primary health care depends for its success on ensuring high-quality care.

In many countries, health care providers and administrators are increasingly concerned about the quality of care. In particular, new methods of treatment are the subjects of studies aiming at developing standard treatment protocols and expected outcomes of treatment for common conditions such as hypertension and cancer. Although these studies make valuable contributions to improving the quality of care, the current approach to the issue has one conspicuous defect. It concentrates almost exclusively on the technical aspects of treatment. It ignores such important issues as overtreatment, iatrogenic disease, the alienation of patients and their families, the unwanted extension of life, and the emotional and financial costs of illness. The present approach sidesteps ethical

84

issues and fosters the belief that only expensive and complex types of treatment and support measures are effective.

All these issues are important in the new concept of health that underlies the regional strategy for health for all. The concept of high-quality care must be extended to cover vital elements of the primary health care approach:

- the effectiveness, safety, efficiency and adequacy of care designed to meet people's needs;

- the acceptability to the users of the services delivered;

- the provision to users of information, their chances for participation, and their satisfaction with services; and

- the protection of service users from unnecessary subjection to expensive, unpleasant, invasive and potentially hazardous equipment, procedures or drugs.

The quality of care is a highly complex subject, requiring much research by multidisciplinary teams representing the biomedical, economic, behavioural and organizational sciences. For this discussion, the concept of the quality of care is broken down into its two major parts: quality assessment and quality assurance.

What is quality?   The first step in quality assessment is a simple question. What is quality? This question can be approached from a technical viewpoint: does care meet professional standards? Another viewpoint is focused on people: does care benefit the person who receives it? The health for all movement clearly takes the second view.

To provide a realistic basis for quality assessment, detailed analyses are needed of the definitions and criteria for high-quality care that prevail among the different groups of people involved in health care delivery. Studies should determine what quality of care means for the users of services (according to their age, sex, social class, state of health, and where they receive care), their families, health professionals (according to specialty, age, sex and where

Priority topics

85

they work), administrators (in hospitals, insurance companies, and rehabilitative and custodial institutions) and the general public.

Studies employing survey and Delphi methods, group discussions, and in-depth interviews could throw light on all the complex aspects of the quality issue. They could also point out converging, as well as conflicting, expectations and interests.

Patterns of care for the same conditions vary considerably among health care providers, health care settings and schools of care. Epidemiological studies are needed to establish what criteria, standards and norms are actually applied in health care. They should determine the patterns of care and detect differences between the professional standards claimed as guides for decisions and the criteria actually employed. Comparative studies are needed to evaluate the quality of the results of different patterns of care.

The psychosocial effects of care are becoming increasingly important aspects of its quality, particularly the aspect known as the art of care. Unfortunately, the assessment of such matters as consumer satisfaction and informed participation in decision-making is still hampered by a serious lack of clear, practical definitions and empirical data. The notion of the art of care must be translated into measurable terms and included in studies on quality assessment.

One special psychosocial aspect of quality of care tends to be easily overlooked: the satisfaction of the providers of care. More studies are needed to assess the psychosocial strain on health professionals giving care in different settings. Studying the strain on family members and other unpaid health workers caring for people at home would be equally important.

The cost-effectiveness of different patterns of care in different health service settings is attracting much attention from politicians, health administrators and the general public. In a way, cost-containment can be considered as a Trojan Horse, smuggling concepts such as positive health, prevention, community participation and teamwork into a city whose inhabitants have been reluctant to consider them. The exact measurement of resources used on a single person or in one element of care is still difficult,

86

however. Studies in health economics are needed to establish standard measures and procedures for detailed assessments of the costs of care in different health care settings.

How to ensure high-quality care.   Once the quality of care can be reliably assessed, the information obtained can be used to improve it or to reduce the cost of care while maintaining a high quality. Audits of quality of care would thus confer a key benefit: they could guide care providers' future decisions. To assist in the making of these decisions, methods must be devised for routinely using the results of quality audits to improve procedures for providing care. This raises complex questions. Is it most effective to transmit information from quality audits on individual care providers, teams, departments or health centres? Should health care teams be measured competitively (against each other) or independently (against their own prior performance)? Recent studies have demonstrated that changing patterns of care can be quite difficult even in uncontroversial clinical areas. Clearly, the tasks of assessing the social and ethical aspects of the provision of health care and establishing mechanisms for quality assurance will be still more complex. Substantial research into organizational behaviour will be needed.

Regional recommendations on the assessment and assurance of the quality of care are not yet well established. Consequently, this may be a good time to encourage countries to set up programmes for quality assessment and assurance.

4

A healthy environment

A healthy physical environment (including homes and work-places) is an important part of positive health. Preventing disease and promoting health by improving the quality of the environment is a new challenge for most Member States of the European Region. It opens new prospects for health policies and health research.

The relationship between environmental pollution and health is an important issue that has attracted new interest in recent decades. The eight targets in this chapter begin with a call for multisectoral policies that protect people from health hazards in the environment (target 18) and for monitoring, assessing and controlling such hazards (target 19). These first two targets are general; one calls for a policy and the other for means of carrying it out. Targets 20–25 address specific issues in environmental health: water pollution, air pollution, food safety, hazardous waste, and risks in the home and the workplace.

All the targets in this group aim not only at protecting people from risks but also at promoting their health through a safe and pleasant environment (the social environment and its effects on health are discussed in Chapter 5). This chapter should therefore be read as a whole whenever Member States decide to use the recommendations in it as a source of inspiration in studying environmental health.

**Knowledge:
the key to action**

Much is known about environmental pollution and the harm it does to health. The environment has deteriorated rapidly in recent decades. Almost every country obviously needs to take more effective action to prevent further damage. The task today is to use available means of monitoring, preventing and controlling pollution, to improve the quality of the environment, including living and working conditions.

Unfortunately, the lack of money often hinders the use of existing knowledge. The funds available do not allow greater use of more comprehensive methods of protecting the environment and human health.

Political and social obstacles also exist. Research into past political decisions for the control of environmental health hazards could show how and why the decisions were made and whether or to what extent they were effective. Research into policy, using the methods of the social and behavioural sciences, must determine what factors impede the use of advances in knowledge. For example, how does health education affect the public?

So far, research has concentrated on gathering knowledge on environmental agents and on people's exposure to them in different settings. While much is known about exposure, little is certain about its effects on health. In particular, much more must be discovered about the effects on human beings of low-dose and long-term exposure. When Member States assign high priority to environmental health, they should give special encouragement to research projects on this topic. Technology in this field is rapidly developing and expanding; it can give valuable aid.

The first step in monitoring, assessing and controlling environmental hazards to health is to understand how environmental pollution produces harmful effects on health.

**The chain
of causes and effects**

Environmental hazards may originate in nature or from human activities. Hazards may arise from physical agents (such as noise and ultrasound, and different kinds of radiation), chemical agents (such as natural cadmium in some areas and pollutants originating

90

from industry and homes) and biological agents (such as viruses, bacteria and other organisms).

Biological agents differ from physical and chemical agents. After being absorbed, a biological agent may multiply and increase the dose. Further, biological agents can adapt themselves to their new environment. They usually cause infectious diseases, but their effects may overlap with those of chemicals. For example, microorganisms may produce toxic chemicals or behave as chemicals after being killed by the host organism in a human body.

Pollution takes the pathways of air, water, soil and food in entering the environment. People can then be exposed to pollution through accidents, incidents or continuous pollution. In accidents, the agent is present in large quantities. The concentration of the agent in an incident, however, is relatively low, although higher than background levels in the environment. Environmental incidents may be associated with, for example, the dumping of waste or areas of intensive industrial activity. Continuous pollution involves exposure to lower concentrations over a long period of time. In all three forms of exposure, the duration of the pollution and the level of contamination are usually inversely related. In addition, the nature of an agent or agents may change in the environment. Little is known, for instance, about how pesticides change after use or their final destination in the environment.

Pollution can affect people in two ways. The first, and probably less important, is a local effect, made when a pollutant touches the human body directly. The second is a systemic effect; after a phase of spread that sometimes changes the nature of the pollutant, the function of an organ or a specific molecule in an organ is affected. This in turn may affect health either immediately or after a number of years.

Exposure to different kinds of agent has different kinds of effect. For example, the effect of a physical agent depends on its nature, the amount of energy, the duration of exposure or absorption and the part of the body exposed. The systemic effects of chemical agents depend on the route of exposure, the amount absorbed, the duration of absorption, the kinetics, biotransformation and excretion of the agent, and the target organ or organs. Exposure usually changes the working of a receptor, an organ or an organ system. Classical toxic effects are visible changes that occur immediately or after some time. In this context, carcinogenicity can be described as an altered functioning of cells, leading after many years to a cancer.

Recent attention has focused on biochemical effects. These are not visible changes in the working of an organ but, for example, alterations in its ability to handle other chemicals. These effects influence the toxic effect of exposure to chemicals. Radioactive chemicals are important topics for study because they are particularly toxic and can harm people in various ways. In addition, the effects of ionizing radiation (a physical agent) must also be studied.

Two ways to define environmental health hazards

The next step in dealing with environmental hazards is to define hazardous situations. This can be done through a two-way approach. First, researchers should study potentially toxic or hazardous agents to determine the risks and effects of exposure. Such effects could include changes in the incidence of disease in communities or groups of people. Second, researchers should investigate effects that may be attributable to environmental contaminants, to identify potentially hazardous agents. Both parts of this approach may help to design policies to prevent or reduce harmful effects on health.

Using the results of research

Practical use of the results of research on environmental health can be made when effects are first defined and then examined for their impact on health. Although people often think that effects are invariably negative, some may be harmless or even desirable.

Further, researchers into environmental health must recognize and consider effects that harm only the environment (although people's wellbeing may be affected in such cases). The difference between assessments of environmental impact and of effects on health must be stressed. Both should be combined in environmental health impact assessments.

Weighting systems are sometimes used to assess the importance of effects on health and thus the need for risk management. For example, priority might be given to a chemical because experiments indicate that it is mutagenic or accumulates in the body. These decisions, however, are usually rather arbitrary.

Eliminating all the risks to health associated with physical, chemical and biological agents, and the disposal of waste is practically impossible. Finding a suitable way to manage risk is thus essential. Such a process should include: risk assessment (identifying hazards and estimating the risks they may pose) and risk evaluation (appraising the possible costs of risks).

Managing environmental risks to health

The result of risk assessment is the establishment of the chain of cause-and-effect relationships. Hazard identification is aimed at agents and risk estimation at the observed effects on people. Risk assessment can be approached from either direction.

The assessment and evaluation of risks should culminate in decisions on how to deal with them. While more or less rational, such decisions are subject to a great variety of pressures. From one side interest groups try to exert influence, while the public presses its opinions, preconceptions and fears from the other.

The decision-maker must evaluate risks, using formal criteria, intuition or an assessment of the balance between the various private and public pressure groups. The decision-maker must also consider people's feelings about taking various kinds of risk. These can vary widely from society to society and from person to person, and depend on a host of cultural, socioeconomic, psychological and time factors, as well as on the type and nature of the risk in question. For example, people may be far more willing to endure risks that they take voluntarily than those imposed on them.

Predictions of risk are made in terms of statistical probabilities, which many people find difficult to visualize and understand. Effective public participation in making decisions about risks requires that the scientific community, industry, the public and decision-makers make a conscious effort to improve communication.

In determining acceptable levels of risk, decision-makers must weigh the public's perception of risk and of the distribution of disadvantages and benefits, along with appraisals of the costs and benefits of various options for risk control. The tools of the social and behavioural sciences are well enough developed to create a data base on the public's perceptions of risk. It may be used to improve the basis for the decision-making process.

In addition, someone has to pay for risk management; economic considerations must be taken fully into account. The cost burden of regulating a risk depends on the options available for controlling it. These options may include forms of self-regulation; for example, a polluter may respond to incentives for assuming the costs of control. Other available methods include insurance against harmful effects. The validity of the economic analysis will depend on the completeness of the data used in risk estimation.

Target 18. Policies for a healthy environment	*By 1990, Member States should have multisectoral policies that effectively protect the environment from health hazards, ensure community awareness and involvement, and support international efforts to curb such hazards affecting more than one country.*

The achievement of this target will require the acceptance by all governments that well coordinated multisectoral efforts are needed at central, regional and local levels, to ensure that human health considerations are regarded as essential prerequisites for industrial and other forms of socioeconomic development, including the introduction of new technologies; the introduction of mechanisms to increase community awareness and involvement in environmental issues with potential implications for human health; and the development of international arrangements for effective control of transfrontier environmental health hazards.

> *By 1990, all Member States should have adequate machinery for the monitoring, assessment and control of environmental hazards which pose a threat to human health, including potentially toxic chemicals, radiation, harmful consumer goods and biological agents.*
>
> *The achievement of this target will require the establishment of well coordinated monitoring programmes with clearly defined objectives; the development of methodologies and health criteria for the assessment of data in relation to control procedures; the investment of adequate levels of funding for control measures, and their introduction and maintenance; and the training and utilization of sufficient numbers of competent personnel for all aspects of environmental health protection.*

**Target 19.
Monitoring, assessment and control of risks in the environment**

Targets 18 and 19 must be discussed together because they share both gaps in knowledge and needs for research. They address environmental health research as a whole and as a background to decision-making and effective risk management.

The task

Target 18 calls for multisectoral policies for a healthy environment and target 19 for the monitoring, assessment and control of environmental hazards that threaten human health, including potentially toxic chemicals (either natural or man-made), radiation, various sources of energy, harmful consumer goods and biological agents. This list is neither exclusive nor comprehensive. The determination of research needs must begin from the establishment of cause-and-effect relationships, not from these examples.

The wording of targets 18 and 19 and the Regional Committee's suggested solutions stress the control of agents as the path to environmental health. This seems misleading in a discussion of research needs. The study of effects is just as important as work on agents.

Studies are needed to collect physical, chemical and biological data as well as data on risk evaluation and risk management. Research is also needed to determine the aim and scope of monitoring,

95

to find ways to keep the public better informed and to encourage people to participate, to study agents and effects, and to develop better methods of risk assessment. More basic research is needed, too.

Priority topics

A clearing-house for data. Many European Member States collect data on environmental agents and risks to health. They record: concentration levels in water, air, soil, food, workplaces and homes; industrial, agricultural and domestic emissions; levels of human exposure and biological contamination or pollution; and findings from monitoring and scientific studies. There are problems, however. In general, information is collected for a variety of purposes. It is sometimes invalid and unreliable, collected in different ways, or not sufficiently comparable. In addition, data on safe levels for human exposure are lacking.

A comprehensive inventory should be made of data on physical, chemical and biological agents, and their effects on the environment and health. It should review the data for their usefulness in preventing environmental risks and protecting health. Such an inventory would be especially helpful in overcoming current difficulties in evaluating the available knowledge of effects on health and the resulting options for risk management. Better predictions of the effects of pollution may also be made. A clearing-house for environmental health data is the best way to build and assess the inventory. To help political decision-makers protect the environment, information on risk evaluation and management should be included. Decision-makers must be able to find information on such topics as:

● the legal and administrative aspects of risk management;

● evaluations of the costs of policy options (including alternative technology);

● the role of fiscal incentives; and

● the public's perceptions of various risks.

Aim and scope of monitoring. Environmental hazards should be monitored to ascertain how and where they should be controlled to

96

prevent harm to health and manage the risk appropriately. This requires an assessment of the whole chain of causes and effects. The next step is to decide, using the assessment, what substances, people and sites should be monitored and how the monitoring should be carried out. Obviously, finding the best solution will depend on the substances given priority and on the people and geographical areas involved. In some cases, the best way of protecting health is to monitor the environment; in others, it is to monitor harmful effects in a population, preferably before symptoms of disease are recognized. Choosing the second option would imply that the agents or pollutants causing a specific effect on health are known, which is rare. In other cases, monitoring must point out the possible causes of a certain effect.

Monitoring must cover effects on the environment and health and, ideally, all aspects of any environmental health risk that require management. In most Member States, monitoring is established in workplaces, to see that maximum admissible concentrations are not exceeded. Similarly, monitoring of the general population usually focuses on maintaining admissible daily intake levels and watching for associated health risks.

So far, exposure to environmental agents in the home has been completely neglected. (Accidents in the home are discussed under target 11, in Chapter 6.) Further, diseases caused by biological agents (such as *Legionella, Pneumocystis, Cryptococcus* and *Toxoplasma* spp.) are becoming more common in the European Region. They are another and perhaps more obvious field for monitoring.

Research is therefore needed to help develop integrated monitoring systems that cover suspected environmental health risks. Suitable ways to assess genetic damage should be included. Research must define what should be monitored and how (through standard procedures for collecting data) if the information is to be of any value for decision-making.

In recent decades, research has focused on ionizing radiation. The methods of assessing the risks of exposure to radiation are well established. The work has led to: the development of the concepts of individual, total and acute doses; the assessment of risks based on the total fuel cycle; analysis of the factors of risks and their combination; knowledge of cellular repair mechanisms; and the development of other concepts used in radiobiology and in protecting people from radiation. These results offer principles and methods that might be useful in monitoring other agents, particularly toxic chemicals. While experts assess risks and design monitoring strategies, they should investigate the applicability of these ideas.

Facts for and action from the public. Everyone should know more about the nature and extent of risks and effective means of protection against them. Such knowledge is particularly important for people who produce risks or are exposed to them, the professionals involved in measuring or dealing with them, and the general public. More knowledge would result in a greater desire for a safe environment. This would encourage decision-makers to try harder to take environmental health fully into account when they plan and assess new socioeconomic development. It is also important to teach health workers about toxicology and convince them that greater knowledge of environmental health will improve the care they provide.

Research should help people to be better informed about and more active in decisions on environmental health issues. This will mean, above all, a search for ways to offer the public opportunities for greater involvement. The behavioural and social sciences can give valuable help in this area.

Questions for basic research. More basic research is needed on environmental health hazards, their causes and possible means of preventing them. Multidisciplinary studies are essential. They must take full advantage of the biomedical and natural sciences. For instance, research to discover people at high risk should have high priority because effective preventive measures should be directed towards those who need them most.

Not everyone who is exposed to particular environmental risks becomes ill. More and more scientists realize that people vary

98

significantly in their susceptibility or resistance to environmental agents. Such variations are to a great extent genetically determined. For example, genetic differences in the efficiency of DNA repair and in the way the metabolism handles harmful foreign substances may contribute to such variability. Genetic damage is particularly serious, since mutagenesis in germ cells may be passed on to future generations. Effects on genes should be studied to prevent disease in susceptible people. Substances that can cause mutations in people and systems for monitoring possible genetic damage are other fruitful topics.

Studies of agents, studies of effects.   In general, more research is needed into how agents interact in the intact animal, in organs and in cellular and subcellular systems. Studies on human volunteers may also be essential in some instances. Important subjects for studies of agents are the interaction of low-dose and long-term exposure to potentially toxic chemicals, and combined exposure to various risks. The biomedical sciences, analytical chemistry, medical toxicology, epidemiology and industrial hygiene must be involved in such research.

Studies of agents that affect health often lack coherence. For example, the effects of a substance that pollutes the environment and perhaps the workplace are studied separately. A combined study of the two areas would allow the analysis of a larger part of the dose–effect relationship.

Studies of effects are needed whenever environmental factors are suspected of causing distinct health effects or changing morbidity patterns. This kind of study has investigated mesotheliomas in insulation workers, emphysema in miners or Itai-Itai disease caused by cadmium pollution. It can reveal the environmental causes of such problems in a relatively short time and thus provide a basis for ways to deal with or prevent them.

Better indicators for assessing risk.   Many agents present at low levels in the environment, especially chemicals, are suspected of harming health only after long-term exposure. So far, there are no indicators to allow researchers to detect such effects at an early stage or to decide how much functional impairment and disability they might cause.

Research is urgently needed in this field. Biological indicators should be developed to detect effects from single agents or combinations of agents. Criteria for diagnosing early changes in a biological system are also needed. Neurobehavioural methods are particularly useful in the study of chemical effects. Effects on groups within the general population (such as children, pregnant women or elderly people) should be studied separately.

Target 20. Control of water pollution

> *By 1990, all people of the Region should have adequate supplies of safe drinking-water, and by the year 1995 pollution of rivers, lakes and seas should no longer pose a threat to human health.*
>
> *The achievement of this target will require, in the less developed countries of the Region, the investment of higher levels of funding for the construction and maintenance of drinking-water supply facilities, with the appropriate mobilization of international and bilateral assistance to reinforce national endeavours, and with the training and utilization of adequate numbers of competent personnel; and in all countries of the Region, the introduction of effective legislative, administrative and technical measures for the surveillance and control of pollution of surface water and groundwater, in order to comply with criteria to safeguard public health.*

The task

Research can help countries protect both fresh and marine water from pollution. In addition, Member States should provide people with safe drinking-water, and conform to the WHO guidelines for drinking-water quality.[a] The treatment of such water is another important topic for research.

---

[a] *Guidelines for drinking-water quality.* Geneva, World Health Organization, 1984, Vol. 1.

Changing agricultural practices. The use of pesticides (insecticides, fungicides and herbicides) in agriculture and forestry has greatly increased in the past few years. The increase will probably continue if nothing is done to stop it. Information seems to be lacking about the damage that the rising use of pesticides does to groundwater, drinking-water and, ultimately, people.

Even when enough knowledge is provided, it probably neither reaches farmers and foresters nor induces them to change their behaviour. These people need to know much more about the harm to the environment and to human beings caused by the overuse of pesticides and fertilizers. They also need incentives to change their agricultural practices. Research in the social and behavioural sciences should satisfy these needs.

Studies on the use of chemicals in agriculture and forestry should be combined with the findings on industrial and household sources of contamination. They should help produce, develop and implement integrated strategies for land-use that will protect water.

Research for safe drinking-water. Nitrates in drinking-water raise particular concern. Almost 30% of the total human intake of nitrates comes from this source. Many European countries exceed the limit of 10 mg nitrate-N per litre set by the WHO guidelines. Unfortunately, this and other such limits for concentrations of substances in drinking-water are based on questionable findings. They do not fully consider the possibility that harmful effects may vary among geographical areas, ethnic groups and cultures.

Carefully designed multidisciplinary studies should be carried out on the toxicity to human beings of pollutants in drinking-water in different countries. These would allow guidelines for drinking-water quality to be adapted to the circumstances in different areas.

Research should also examine the treatment of drinking-water. Better knowledge of the health effects of organic and inorganic compounds in water is needed; so is appropriate technology for protecting water sources. Further, drinking-water resources are becoming so scarce that it is increasingly necessary to use water from contaminated sources. The physical, chemical and biological methods of removing contaminants from water require further study. Special attention must be paid to finding better and more cost-effective methods for purifying water; many are still experimental.

**Target 21.
Protection against
air pollution**

> *By 1995, all people of the Region should be effectively protected against recognized health risks from air pollution.*
>
> *The achievement of this target will require the introduction of effective legislative, administrative and technical measures for the surveillance and control of both outdoor and indoor air pollution, in order to comply with criteria to safeguard human health.*

The task

The Regional Committee's solutions for achieving this target stress the need to strengthen measures to control indoor air pollution, as well as emissions from industry, motor vehicles, agriculture and homes. Research has a particularly important role in the development of new air quality guidelines and the prevention of atmospheric pollution across national frontiers.

Priority topics

Health hazards of indoor air pollution. While scientists, politicians and the public have concentrated on industrial and motor vehicle emissions, health hazards from homes and indoor air pollutants have been largely ignored. Establishing an integrated data base on air pollutants is an important task for research. Special consideration should be given to using the data to increase people's awareness of potentially health-damaging air pollutants indoors and of the influence of insulation on ventilation and pollution. Studies should also examine the relationship between

102

outdoor and indoor pollution. Another subject deserving attention is pollution inside automobiles.

New guidelines for air quality. Monitoring in most parts of the European Region has been restricted to atmospheric pollutants such as sulfuric oxides and particulate matter, nitrogen oxides and oxidants, hydrocarbons and ozone. The Regional Office for Europe has produced new air quality guidelines[a] that include air pollutants not previously covered by surveillance systems. The new guidelines also consider air pollutants with indirect effects on health. For example, metals settle on the soil and may contaminate the environment and damage health. The degree to which such air pollutants affect the environment and health should be assessed.

Air pollution across national boundaries. Transfrontier air pollution poses serious problems. The acidification of lakes and rivers has harmed fauna and flora in the Region, particularly in northern Europe. Some evidence points to nitrogen oxides, sulfuric oxides and ammonia as the causes of the damage, although the causes are not yet clearly understood. In particular, researchers should discover more about the effect of toxic metals such as mercury and aluminium on the soil and ecosystem.

Research in this field must be stepped up. Coordinated and interdisciplinary studies are required on the causes of transfrontier air pollution and possible ways of controlling it. The spread of radionuclides from one country to another should also be considered, since the accident to the nuclear power plant at Chernobyl has demonstrated that the current measures for control need improvement.

---

[a] *Air quality guidelines for Europe.* Copenhagen, WHO Regional Office for Europe, 1987 (WHO Regional Publications, European Series, No. 23).

**Target 22.
Food safety**

> *By 1990, all Member States should have significantly reduced health risks from food contamination and implemented measures to protect consumers from harmful additives.*
>
> *The achievement of this target will require the introduction of effective legislative, administrative and technical measures for the surveillance and control of food contamination at all stages of production, distribution, storage, sale and use; and the implementation of measures to control the use of harmful food additives.*

The task
Studies are needed to examine new methods of handling food and to find better ways to inform people about food hygiene.

Priority topics
Investigating food handling. As a result of new industrial techniques and changes in people's lifestyles (and thus in their patterns of food consumption) food handling has changed a great deal in recent years. The effects of these changes on health are not clear. Research should investigate the production and storage techniques used by the food industry and how consumers store and prepare food in their homes. Do these practices harm health?

Keeping the public informed. People should know more about food hygiene. Education on the topic should start in primary school, to change the attitudes of the public towards health hazards related to food.

Changing attitudes and behaviour is difficult (see Chapter 5). Educational programmes on the actual risks associated with food must be developed and their effectiveness carefully evaluated. Sociological and psychological knowledge about attitude and behavioural changes must be used in programme development.

While the public must learn, food producers must act. The target specifies the surveillance and control of food contamination as their responsibilities.

104

Target 23.
Protection from
hazardous wastes

> *By 1995, all Member States should have eliminated major known health risks associated with the disposal of hazardous wastes.*
>
> *The achievement of this target will require the introduction of effective legislative, administrative and technical measures for the surveillance and control of hazardous wastes; and the introduction of effective measures to eliminate health risks due to previously dumped wastes.*

The task

The chemical industry is the main producer of hazardous waste. Protecting health from the risks it poses will necessitate special regulatory and administrative procedures. Although hazardous waste makes up a relatively small percentage of all the waste produced by industry, agriculture and households, its disposal has contaminated dumping sites. These in turn are important sources of pollution in soil and underground water.

Technical measures to handle, transport or treat chemical waste are considered to be the responsibility of industry. Legal and administrative measures must aim at ensuring that industry shoulders the burden. The same principle, of course, also applies to other types of waste, such as nuclear waste.

Research can assess the damage done to health by hazardous chemical waste. Studies can also help supply answers to important questions about the continued development of low-waste and non-waste industrial techniques and disposal methods.

Priority topics

The effects of hazardous waste on health. Serious problems arise from the final disposal of non-treatable chemical waste. It may result in the long-term exposure of people and their environment to harmful chemicals. No one has yet devised a completely safe way to dispose of hazardous waste.

Determining the types of hazardous waste that are especially harmful to the general public and the workers involved in its disposal (because of the quantity and/or toxicity of waste) is a first step in developing a safe disposal method. The effects of hazardous waste on health must be assessed; methods for comprehensive

105

analyses of the most dangerous types should be developed. Mathematical models could be powerful tools in this task.

Creating less waste and better ways to dispose of it. Technical measures to safeguard health should include low-waste and non-waste techniques, safer methods of physicochemical, thermal and microbiological disposal, and means of eliminating risks from new and existing dumps.

Low-waste and non-waste technology aims at helping industry to eliminate or reduce the amount of waste produced, by reusing it in the process that generated it and producing waste that may be used for other purposes (as secondary raw materials, fertilizers or energy). These techniques also offer possibilities for changes in production: the replacement and pretreatment of raw materials, the replacement of products and the separation of waste into streams for treatment. More research is needed to establish how and how much low-waste and non-waste technology and disposal methods can reduce risks.

Target 24. Healthy homes

> *By the year 2000, all people of the Region should have a better opportunity of living in houses and settlements which provide a healthy and safe environment.*
>
> *The achievement of this target will require the acceleration of programmes of housing construction and improvement; the development of international health criteria for housing, space, heating, lighting, disposal of wastes, noise control and safety, while taking into account the special needs of groups such as young families, the elderly and the disabled; legislative, administrative and technical measures to comply with such criteria; the improvement of community planning in order to enhance health and wellbeing by improving traffic safety, providing open spaces and recreational areas, and facilitating human interaction, etc.; and the equipment of all dwellings with proper sanitation facilities and the provision of sewers and an adequate public cleansing and wastes collection and disposal system in all human settlements of sufficient size.*

Further research is urgently needed to determine the consequences of bad housing on human wellbeing and the effects on health of the home environment.

Hazards of bad housing. The criteria and standards recommended by WHO for the development of urban areas have often been neglected. Towns have grown haphazardly and shanty towns have sprung up, particularly in the Mediterranean area.

Some of the consequences for health of bad housing (such as those resulting from inadequate sanitation) are well known. Others (particularly the psychosocial aspects of the urban environment) are often neglected or still unclear. City dwellers may have to cope with, for instance, overcrowding, anxiety about the risk of violence, and large-scale housing projects in which it is difficult to know their neighbours and which therefore lead to isolation.

How can such factors harm some people's health? An inventory of the psychosocial factors that may damage health should be drawn up. Community planners could use it as a source of necessary information and to assess effects on health.

The home environment. More knowledge is needed on the health effects of various environmental factors in homes and of physical variables (such as temperature, humidity, lighting, insulation, air movement, noise and ventilation).

The effects of radon are another important topic for research. The inhalation of radon in mines has been shown to cause lung cancer. To assess the effects of radon in the home, epidemiological studies should investigate its effects in conjunction with those of other pollutants.

Yet another agent that deserves further research is noise. The world, especially the urban parts of it, has become a much louder place. So far, only individual sources of noise have been studied. Studies on the effects of multiple sources of noise (from the home, leisure pursuits, the workplace, air traffic and ground transport) would provide additional information useful in the design of control measures.

**Target 25.
Healthy
working conditions**

> *By 1995, people of the Region should be effectively protected against work-related health risks.*
>
> *The achievement of this target will require the introduction of appropriate occupational health services to cover the needs of all workers; the development of health criteria for the protection of workers against biological, chemical and physical hazards; the implementation of technical and educational measures to reduce work-related risk factors; and the safeguarding of specially vulnerable groups of workers.*

Priority topics

The quality of occupational health services. Ensuring that occupational health services cover all places of work, including the home, deserves high priority. With few exceptions, occupational health services are not available to large sections of the working population, such as farmers or employees in small businesses. Even when services are provided — usually for industrial workers — monitoring is often insufficient. Accidents at work remain an important cause of disability and death. Statistics do not provide a full picture of all the diseases related to work (see target 11, in Chapter 6).

Evaluation should always follow the introduction or expansion of occupational health services. Because coordinating these services with other forms of health care is also important, the evaluation of occupational services must be a part of research on primary health care (see Chapter 3). Like other kinds of health care, occupational services should be examined for equity, effectiveness and impact. In addition, the studies should show the extent to which the services conform to international conventions such as those approved by the International Labour Organisation.

Improved guidelines for occupational exposure. Countries should cooperate more closely on limits for occupational exposure (maximum admissible concentration levels and biological tolerance levels), including guidelines for safety measures. Member States should also try to harmonize their guidelines as much as possible. The limits on exposure to toxic chemicals recommended by national and international bodies are still hotly debated.

The effects of a changing work environment. Special research questions are raised by the introduction of new technology in the workplace. Data processing and automatic control systems, for example, are changing the rhythm, tasks and responsibilities of work. Studies should investigate the physical and psychosocial effects of the changing work environment, to design measures for handling and preventing them, if necessary.

Such studies require the close collaboration of experts in occupational health, the biomedical sciences, the social and behavioural sciences, public health and environmental health. The lack of such collaboration has led to duplication of studies. It is also largely responsible for the occasionally poor quality or the lack of methodological rigour of past studies.

5

Healthy lifestyles

The chapters on appropriate care and a healthy environment covered two of the kinds of change necessary for health for all. This chapter discusses the third. The regional strategy for health for all explicitly recognizes that people's lifestyles strongly influence their health. Unfortunately, a lifestyle does not result solely from one person's free choice. Societal and environmental factors also shape the lifestyles prevailing in a society and the groups within it, opening exciting vistas of using lifestyles to improve health. How can this be done?

Targets 13–17 address the challenge of improving health by promoting healthy ways of living, and form a neatly dovetailed unit. Target 13 calls on Member States to make policies to promote healthy lifestyles and to ensure community participation in the work. The other targets detail four parts of such a policy: programmes for social support, programmes to increase people's ability to maintain their health, increases in health-enhancing behaviour, and decreases in health-damaging behaviour.

This subject obviously requires that the social and behavioural sciences contribute to research on lifestyles and health.

Three caveats

Again, people's behaviour is the result not simply of free personal choice but of the structure of society, pressures from the groups to which they belong, and conditioning in prevailing patterns of thinking, feeling and acting. The room for the personal choice of

111

behaviour is severely limited and difficult to determine in individual cases. In research on lifestyles, the primary aim of the social sciences is to point out the factors in society that affect health-related patterns of behaviour. These factors include working and living conditions, expectations and conflicts arising from the roles that society imposes on people, the influence of interest groups, and questions of power and authority in society. Any attempt to understand or to change health-related patterns of behaviour requires the study of the people concerned and, probably far more important, the societal factors that shape their behaviour.

Further, the social and behavioural sciences share a characteristic that distinguishes them from the natural sciences. The objects of study in the social and behavioural sciences are subjects, just as researchers or health planners are subjects. They are human beings with as much consciousness, freedom and dignity as anyone who tries to analyse and influence their behaviour. The first step in trying to understand and perhaps to change other people's behaviour must therefore be to analyse its meaning to the people who practise it. Otherwise, any attempt to change the behaviour is bound to miss its mark. This analysis will call for the use of both quantitative and qualitative research methods (such as participant observation, comprehensive interviews, group discussions of problems, and field research).

Finally, a person establishes a pattern of behaviour because the behaviour serves a purpose for the individual and for society. In most instances, the influence on health is a side effect. Even when people claim that health is among their highest-ranking values, other values (such as personal and collective achievement and prestige, economic success and emotional satisfaction) often take higher priority in everyday life. People pursue these even at the expense of their health. Any attempt to change health-damaging behaviour will thus have two requirements for success. First, researchers must analyse the primary purposes of the behaviour at both individual and collective levels. Second, the alternatives proposed must fulfil these purposes as well as promote health.

112

Research into lifestyles and health obviously requires close inter-disciplinary cooperation between the biomedical and the social and behavioural sciences. In addition, research into the various disciplines connected with the allied health professions is an essential component of a comprehensive scientific approach to lifestyles and health. These disciplines could probably mediate between the biomedical and behavioural sciences because they employ the theory and practice of both.

Although there are examples of well functioning interdisciplinary research, combining different scientific approaches remains difficult. People with different academic backgrounds, notions of research and experience must be persuaded to work together with mutual understanding. Research workers must also agree on a division of labour that leads to specific, integrated answers to the questions posed rather than scattered and separate findings. In addition, the question of research methods may cause some difficulty in interdisciplinary research projects. Although the effects of lifestyles on health call for a combination of various quantitative and qualitative methods, combining the results yielded by different methods into a coherent and useful whole may pose considerable problems.

Interdisciplinary research is so important and complex that it should also be a topic for study. Research could help to solve the methodological, organizational and sociopsychological problems involved by determining:

- the nature of the obstacles and where they occur;

- the characteristics of examples of successful cooperation and the prerequisites for repeating their success; and

- whether other institutions or sectors in health could benefit from the same approach.

Further, students in the sciences related to health should be prepared for interdisciplinary cooperation. For example, under-graduates could be offered introductory courses on other disciplines. Postgraduate students could receive extended basic training

The linchpin: interdisciplinary research

113

in these disciplines (see target 36, Chapter 2). All should learn that different aspects of a subject call for different scientific approaches and methods of research.

Themes in lifestyles research

The four themes of lifestyles research discussed here indicate topics and goals of research that can make particularly valuable contributions to improving this important factor in health.

Studying lifestyles

A lifestyle may be described as a cluster of closely interrelated behaviour patterns that depend on social and economic conditions, education, age and many other factors. At present, scientific evidence is often lacking on different types of lifestyle, their components, their distribution in the population and the factors that determine them. The first step in assessing the effects of different lifestyles on health is obtaining sufficient knowledge of the lifestyles themselves. Therefore, developing indicators of lifestyles and establishing a constantly updated information base on prevalent lifestyles are essential and urgent tasks.

The regional lifestyle indicators mainly cover well established forms of health-damaging behaviour. Research into appropriate indicators of lifestyles is urgently needed. Studies should assess present indicators and discover what new indicators are needed and how to measure them. Finally, the indicators should be applied throughout the Region, for eventual use in comparative research. Thorough qualitative studies are needed to obtain the background information on which valid and reliable quantitative indicators can be based.

Because lifestyles change, indicators should be sensitive to changes in health-related behaviour. Traditional surveys focus on behaviour or statements about behaviour at discrete moments in time. They do not reflect the process of change; nor are they appropriate for the study of communities rather than aggregated individuals.

New measures and new techniques of data collection are needed. These requirements emphasize the importance of regional studies and of community participation both in intervention programmes and in the accompanying research projects. Research projects must remain in close contact with the target groups of the programmes, to observe and monitor changes in behaviour in a valid and reliable way.

In addition, the present infrastructure for research into lifestyles is inadequate. It should be improved in three ways. First, long-term interdisciplinary research groups need to be established on a regional level. The continuity of work can be assured if a core group has a permanent source of funds. Second, the allied health professions should be encouraged to do more research. These professionals could perform independent studies or participate in interdisciplinary work. Third, the members of committees that review proposals for research on lifestyles should include people experienced in the theories and methods of social and behavioural sciences. This will allow all aspects of the proposals to be properly assessed.

How do genetic factors affect the relationship between lifestyles and health? This question prompts two others for research.

Genetics and lifestyles

- How do individual genetic conditions influence the health effect of a lifestyle?

- Do genetic conditions influence lifestyles themselves or certain types of behaviour?

More basic research could answer the first question. The health effects of a given type of behaviour vary considerably among different people. For example, not all heavy smokers develop lung cancer, and obesity or lack of physical exercise does not always lead to cardiovascular problems. Obviously, health and behaviour are indirectly connected through intermediary variables. It seems reasonable to assume that genetic differences are one of these variables. Scientific evidence for this relationship, however, is still scarce. More detailed knowledge is needed. If genetic conditions predispose certain people to adverse health effects from certain types of behaviour, risk groups could be defined much more precisely and could probably be influenced more easily.

The second question is undoubtedly much more controversial. Nevertheless, in some instances, evidence seems to show that genetic conditions are connected to lifestyle. Individual differences in basal metabolism, for example, might very well explain differences in eating habits. Different recommendations on adequate nutrition would be made in such cases.

Despite the difficulties, genetic influences on health-related behaviour deserve further, preferably interdisciplinary, research.

AIDS   The recent upsurge of AIDS, a new infectious disease, has awakened people to the close relationship between lifestyles and health. AIDS shows a direct and conspicuous connection between behaviour and damage to health.

There is no cure. Only prevention can protect people against the disease. The success of preventive measures depends largely on people's sense of responsibility for their own health and that of others. Since AIDS is a sexually transmitted disease, the importance of healthy sexual behaviour to a healthy lifestyle is brought into sharp focus. Further, the threat of AIDS is likely to have a profound effect on the nature and forms of sexual relations in the high-risk groups and the general population.

The deadly nature of AIDS gives urgency to the need for intensified research into the aspects of the disease that are related to lifestyles (see also target 5 in Chapter 6). Many topics deserve high priority. How much do the general population and groups within it know about AIDS? How much does the information provided actually change behaviour? What measures can increase people's sense of responsibility for their health and for the health of others? Can some measures reduce the risk of spreading the disease in the population without discriminating against certain high-risk groups?

The goal: health promotion   The kernel of the lifestyles approach and of targets 13–17 is the intention to change prevailing lifestyles: to spread health-enhancing

116

lifestyles and reduce those that damage health. Attempts to make healthy lifestyles the normal way of life in a society pose six general problems that affect the content and methods of the research needed.

First, the concept of positive health means a complete change of paradigm in the scientific approach to health. Shifting the focus of scientific inquiry from the causes of illness to the causes of health is highly promising and intellectually exciting. At present, however, this new approach has only begun to be defined and tested. The scientific community should take up the promotion of this new concept from WHO. Research into all aspects of positive health should be encouraged.

The concept of positive health is also an integral part of other targets. Gains in positive health can be expected to result from healthier lifestyles, a healthier environment and more effective systems of health care. This overlap points up the difficulties in identifying the separate parts of positive health. It is also the reason for the overlap in recommendations for research on positive health.

Second, a legitimate wish to influence other people's lifestyles for their own benefit must be balanced against their basic right to choose their own ways of life. This can be done only if the people subjected to an intervention have an equal say in planning and running the intervention programme and the related research projects. Current means of community participation — essential to any programme — are unsatisfactory.

Third, promoting healthy lifestyles, if carried to extremes, could lead to the danger of healthism (establishing an ideal of a healthy, fully socially integrated, and psychologically well balanced person as a social norm). Physical and emotional suffering, loneliness, poverty, misery, illness and death will remain parts of the human condition.

Adopting the ideal of a healthy person as a norm could help many people to choose healthy lifestyles. On the other hand, it could push everyone who did not meet the norm to the margins of society. This could be avoided if a realistic concept were developed that combined the thrust of health for all with the facts of suffering, illness and death in every human life. Public discussion is the only solution to this issue. Health research could provide the material to stimulate such discussion.

Fourth, some groups (Alcoholics Anonymous, Weightwatchers, people with coronary heart disease and self-help and mutual-aid groups) seem to succeed in promoting health. These groups share certain features. They provide their members with social reinforcement and integration into everyday life, and with the chance to participate in planning and running the groups' activities. The groups' success suggests that these features encourage people to make permanent changes in their behaviour.

Health promotion programmes in general would probably benefit if ways of introducing such factors into other forms of health promotion could be explored, tested and evaluated.

Fifth, intervention programmes that focus exclusively on well established forms of risk behaviour (such as excessive smoking, alcohol abuse and overeating) can easily lead to moralistic attitudes, including victim-blaming. These impose an extra burden on people already at increased risk. To avoid these attitudes, a concept should be developed that reconciles personal responsibility with external influences on individual risk behaviour.

Hitherto, health promotion has attempted to exert a direct influence on the behaviour of individuals. At least equal weight should be given, however, to attempts to change the occupational and social factors that condition behaviour related to health. This issue is complex and socially and politically sensitive. Nevertheless, more intensive basic research should be done on the possibilities of changing the structure of the world of work and of society as a whole.

Sixth, programmes for health promotion require careful evaluation. Such programmes provide a good deal of information about health to influence people's attitudes, beliefs and intentions. Very little is yet known, however, about how or whether these changes affect behaviour or health.

Research into health promotion must determine whether intervention programmes actually cause changes in lifestyle and whether

118

such changes improve people's health. Above all, evaluative studies could help to find the most promising measures and conditions for change in different groups of people. Research could thus lead to the selection of specific programmes for specific target groups. Because evaluation requires a great deal of time, money and personnel, it may be sufficient to conduct detailed evaluative studies on model or demonstration programmes. The results could then be used to decide whether the programmes should be expanded.

By 1990, national policies in all Member States should ensure that legislative, administrative and economic mechanisms provide broad intersectoral support and resources for the promotion of healthy lifestyles and ensure effective participation of the people at all levels of such policy-making.

The attainment of this target could be significantly supported by strategic health planning at cabinet level, to cover broad intersectoral issues that affect lifestyle and health, the periodic assessment of existing policies in their relationship to health, and the establishment of effective machinery for public involvement in policy planning and development.

**Target 13.
Healthy public policy**

Although policy is the province of policy-makers, research can give valuable support to the people making healthy public policies.

The task

Monitoring policy development. National policies should be continuously and comprehensively monitored to determine whether they are actually being implemented. These policies may include tax policies designed to discourage the consumption of harmful substances, regulation of the subsidies given for the manufacture of food and other products, measures to protect consumers, regulations on the advertising of harmful products, and legislative action aimed at reducing inequities in health.

Priority topics

Studies of policy issues should determine the effectiveness of existing health-related legislation and regulations. Progress reports should be prepared at regular intervals. The publication of such reports should help to develop appropriate policies. Comparisons between countries are likely to provide additional aid. An analytical model should be developed to facilitate comprehensive analysis and comparisons; it should systematically single out important policy issues and allow the assessment of existing policies.

Assessing policies and programmes designed to change harmful working and living conditions is particularly important. Analyses are also needed of policies and programmes aimed at shifting production from harmful products (such as habit-forming substances, weapons and polluting vehicles) to healthy goods and services (particularly healthy foods).

Obstacles to healthy lifestyles. Research must determine how laws, regulations or policies raise obstacles to healthy lifestyles. All policies that affect health should be reviewed. These reviews should extend beyond the policies intended to affect health (whether directly or indirectly) to those with unintended consequences for health.

Research should seek the most important obstacles to achieving the target in good time, such as laws and regulations that limit public access to health knowledge or health records. Other hindrances may result from the opposition of pressure groups to adequate legislation on, for instance, family planning and sexual education.

Obstacles may also arise from policies in other sectors aimed at, for example, income maintenance, food services and housing. The side effects of such policies may damage people's ability to function, opportunities for social integration and support, and chances to support and care for family members. Policies hindering the attainment of target 13 may include public subsidies that maintain or even increase the production of harmful substances. Pricing policies may limit people's access to healthy food and promote unhealthy eating patterns. Agricultural, livestock and manufacturing practices may limit the ability to choose healthy types of food, free of hormones and antibiotics. Realistic research into such policies must also analyse their primary purposes and propose alternative means of fulfilling them.

A lack of indicators is a particularly important obstacle to the achievement of target 13. Behavioural data, even on the harmful practices that have been studied most extensively (smoking and excessive alcohol consumption), are often lacking. Without reliable and valid measures, sensitive to changes in health-related behaviour, finding out whether policies actually change behaviour is impossible.

Lifestyle indicators should therefore be included in periodic national health surveys. If scientifically designed and analysed, the surveys could provide a great deal more than purely descriptive information at little extra cost. Researchers could use statistical procedures and analytical models to analyse causal processes and chains of influence in complex health data. In addition, existing data from such sources as sickness funds and health insurance schemes should be examined for information related to lifestyles. Much could be obtained if existing data were analysed in new ways (see target 35, Chapter 2). For example, national data on household expenditure, used for the assessment of dietary profiles, could also be the basis for planning a nutrition policy.

Community participation.   Studies are needed to assess whether or to what degree the people concerned have a say in health-related legislation and programme planning. Communities could be measured against an ideal healthy community, to allow the analysis of communities' health resources, to point out health-enhancing policies, gaps in policies, and factors that interfere with the effective development and use of these resources. Comparative evaluations could be made of existing models of community participation in health care and health promotion. Such studies would assess their effectiveness and possibilities for use in other settings.

People's attitudes towards and priorities for health are aspects of public participation. These perceptions should be studied and assessed for their influence on the development of policies that affect health.

Target 14.
Social support
systems

> **By 1990, all Member States should have specific programmes which enhance the major roles of the family and other social groups in developing and supporting healthy lifestyles.**
>
> *The attainment of this target could be significantly supported by establishing close intersectoral links between health and social welfare programmes, primarily at the local level, and by securing funds for projects that enhance joint community action.*

The task   Some aspects of lifestyle are either important prerequisites for healthy lifestyles or essential parts of them. People with healthy lifestyles have:

● sufficient social support, especially in dealing with crises or chronic problems;

● appropriate ways to solve problems, resolve conflicts and make decisions, and an ability to think for themselves; and

● an ability to look after their own health, to evaluate symptoms and to make decisions about health care.

All three of these are highly important. They need further definition, and their impact on health and behaviour should be analysed. In addition, indicators that allow the assessment of social support and coping capacities should be developed.

Priority topics   *Social support.*   Social support works in two ways. People's social networks — families, friends, colleagues, peers and others — shape their attitudes and behaviour, and support them in times of trouble.
   People's integration into social networks affects their health and shapes health-related behaviour; in this sense, a term such as social integration or the influence of social networks might be more

122

accurate than social support. Social networks may both help and harm people's health. On the one hand, families, households, peer groups, neighbours and working groups may very well buffer their members against stress. On the other hand, social networks create and perpetuate severe conflicts in many cases, with all their negative influences on health. Social integration in itself is not necessarily a healthy element in a lifestyle.

Much more must be known about social networks if intervention programmes to strengthen their positive influences are to succeed. For example, what is the relative importance of different social networks at different stages in life? What are the effects of different types of family and group structures on the health and behaviour of their members?

Special attention should be paid to the impact of changes in family and household structures, in parents' and children's roles, in the role expectations imposed on women and men, in patterns of authority and the structure and functions of peer groups at school, and in work and leisure activities. A detailed analysis of the influences of social networks on starting and maintaining health-damaging patterns of behaviour, especially during adolescence, is particularly important. Health surveys and case studies could be used to examine the factors associated with a change, or failure to change, to healthier lifestyles in young adulthood and at other ages.

In a narrower sense, social support means emotional and material care for people who are facing difficult problems. Increasing evidence shows that adequate social support gives significant protection to people confronted with severe crises or long-term problems. Nevertheless, many questions require more detailed answers from empirical studies.

- What is the relative importance of material and emotional support to healthy lifestyles? How can the family — as opposed to other parts of the network — effectively meet various needs for support? What factors determine the relationship between received support and perceived support?

- What criteria make it possible to distinguish the supportive from the destructive influences of social relations?

- Does social support have a direct effect on health? Or does its role as a buffer against stress help to protect health indirectly?

- Under what circumstances can professional services actually fill gaps in a social network?

Coping. Chronic conflict and stress can be considered to have major effects on health. Enhancing people's capacity to cope with them is thus an important element in healthy lifestyles.

At present, scientific knowledge of coping mechanisms (such as those for coping with cancer) is similar to that of social support; it is sufficient to prove that they affect health. Many questions, however, call for more decisive answers from research.

- How does coping capacity depend on people's material resources?

- Do specific problems call for specific coping strategies? Or is a positive attitude (active confrontation and fighting spirit — not passive resignation, denial or avoidance — or a personal sense that life is worth living in all circumstances) towards all problems more effective?

- What criteria can be used to distinguish between more or less successful coping strategies? Does a person cope better by using one particularly successful strategy or several strategies, applied as aspects of a problem change?

- Do characteristics such as education, social stratum, sex, religious affiliation and age affect people's ability to cope?

- To what extent and in what ways are styles of coping related to personality (and therefore relatively resistant to induced change)? How far are they simply patterns of socially learnt behaviour (which can be changed)?

124

- Does social support benefit health indirectly by aiding the development of effective coping strategies?

- Can people gain special coping abilities in self-help and mutual-aid groups?

Making decisions about health. If social support is to work well, people must be able to assess their own condition and to ask for help if they need it. Physical, mental or psychological symptoms are usually interpreted first by the person who experiences them. The person assesses the severity of the symptoms and decides whether lay or professional care is needed. Social networks strongly influence these interpretations.

Research topics should include how these processes differ among social strata and age groups, the role of social networks, the non-rational factors that influence decisions and lead to underuse or overuse of professional services, and how the professional care system can strengthen or weaken people's capacity and willingness to make decisions about their own health.

How can people retain this power of decision within the professional health care system? This question, on a rather sensitive subject, sparks off other questions for research.

- When does the legitimate authority of the health professional actually leave room for lay participation in choosing among diagnostic, therapeutic and rehabilitative procedures (for example, mastectomy as opposed to local excision in breast cancer)?

- What factors influence the capacity and willingness of professionals to encourage the users of services to take part in decision-making?

- How much do patients actually participate in decision-making in health care settings? Do public and private health care systems differ in this respect?

125

Support for support programmes. Several types of programme are recommended to help families and social networks support and care for their members. For example, professional support services should be offered to families in the community. These services could provide child care, complement the care of ill or disabled members in the family, and give advice to help resolve conflicts. In addition, programmes in the local community should mobilize social support for especially vulnerable groups, such as elderly people living alone, the disabled, migrants and single parents with young children. Finally, health education programmes should be directed at social networks, in which people learn their health behaviour. Since people adopt many patterns of behaviour early in life, special attention should be paid to the influence of social networks on children and adolescents.

Research could support the planning and successful implementation of such programmes in several ways. Community-based studies should assess the need for special programmes. The evaluation of programmes and comparison of different models would point out the most promising approaches. In addition, new models should be developed, tested and evaluated on the basis of recent research findings on social support, coping and decision-making.

**Target 15.
Knowledge
and motivation
for healthy behaviour**

> *By 1990, educational programmes in all Member States should enhance the knowledge, motivation and skills of people to acquire and maintain health.*
>
> *The attainment of this target could be significantly supported by ensuring an adequate and effective infrastructure and funding for health education programmes at all levels.*

The task   Health education is a path to achieving this target. Again, current practices in health education tend to provide people with information intended to affect their attitudes, beliefs and intentions. Very little is known about the effects of changes in knowledge on behaviour. Evaluative research should thus establish criteria for judging, first, whether behaviour changes as a result of new information, and then whether these changes affect health. Research into several areas could help people improve their health.

Places, people and subjects for health education. Formal education systems, by transmitting cultural values and expectations in addition to knowledge, have great influence in the shaping of perceptions, attitudes and behaviour. The greatest contribution to achieving all five lifestyle targets may lie in giving children an understanding of the importance of establishing a healthy lifestyle. The basic school system is an essential resource in this task. If it is used effectively, people skilled in teaching and educational psychology can impart knowledge and motivation for healthy behaviour in a natural setting. Case studies and demonstration projects could help to find promising ways of integrating education on lifestyles into all school curricula. A special topic for study would be teachers' attitudes towards health.

Families, peer groups and colleagues are probably even more powerful than schools in shaping lifestyles. People usually spend most of their time in one or another of these groups. In the course of everyday life, such groups transmit the value accorded to health, nutritional patterns, attitudes towards sex and family planning, the assessment of tolerable risks, and many other attitudes and types of behaviour. Research should describe and analyse the content and processes of informal health education in these groups. How do they affect health behaviour? Studies should test and evaluate the chances of influencing them in a positive way.

Even when lifestyle education is generally adopted, special programmes and campaigns for health education will still be needed. The development of community health information systems, adapted to local conditions, could be a particularly promising approach. Research could help by analysing programmes for health promotion and health education in communities from inception to implementation. Studies should evaluate the programmes,

Priority topics

127

examining: public attitudes at the outset of the programmes, means of community participation, differences in the effectiveness of programmes with different kinds of organization or funding, and changes in public attitudes and behaviour in the course of the programmes. The reasons for failing to obtain community participation or to change behaviour should also be investigated.

All health education programmes should give special attention to healthy nutrition (see target 16). Research could support such programmes through studies of basic nutritional patterns, their subjective meaning, and the acceptability of proposed changes in diet to different social groups.

Obstacles to health education. Once established, coping behaviour and lifestyle patterns are difficult to modify. Studies are needed to determine how people receive and use information on health at various stages in life. Small-scale action research projects and case studies are probably the best means of finding the obstacles to knowledge and motivation for healthy behaviour.

Detailed analyses are needed to determine how certain external factors affect the behaviour of individuals. These factors include: advertising campaigns (which play on the themes of maturity, independence, strength and beauty to promote harmful products), the sponsorship of sporting events by companies that produce health-damaging products, peer pressure, and blocked opportunities or limited options in the environment.

When a person receives contradictory messages from industry and from health education, the second suffers. Social factors that hamper health education should be considered from several viewpoints. People should be helped to resist these well organized attacks on their health behaviour. Such obstacles must be clearly identified and tackled through political action such as legislation or taxation. Comparative studies could then evaluate the effects of such measures on behaviour and health.

Another obstacle to health education is the lack of coordination between agencies and groups within and outside government. Research could help these groups work together on programmes and campaigns. Studies could help to initiate and ease such cooperation by analysing the aims and methods of the groups and organizations active in health education, determining the obstacles to closer cooperation, and exploring ways of overcoming them.

Health education in health care. One of the most important arenas for health education is the health care system. Relatively little is yet known about how its structure and personnel influence people's knowlege of and motivation for healthy behaviour. Two kinds of research are urgently needed. First, descriptive analyses should be made of what actually happens in general practitioners' offices, hospitals and outpatient clinics, homes for the elderly, psychiatric hospitals, institutions for the mentally ill, and rehabilitation centres. How do these events influence people's behaviour? The influences resulting from the lifestyles of care providers and health educators deserve particular attention. Second, comparative evaluations should be made of different ways of organizing health care systems, to single out those that can contribute most to health education.

<table>
<tr><td>

By 1995, in all Member States, there should be significant increases in positive health behaviour, such as balanced nutrition, nonsmoking, appropriate physical activity and good stress management.

This could be achieved if clear targets in these areas were set in each Member State, e.g. a minimum of 80% of the population as nonsmokers and a 50% reduction in national tobacco consumption, and if steps were taken by WHO and other international organizations to promote cooperation in health promotion activities throughout the Region in order to make a wider impact on basic health values.

</td><td>

**Target 16.
Promoting positive
health behaviour**

</td></tr>
</table>

**Target 17.
Decreasing
health-damaging
behaviour**

> *By 1995, in all Member States, there should be significant de-creases in health-damaging behaviour, such as overuse of alcohol and pharmaceutical products; use of illicit drugs and dangerous chemical substances; and dangerous driving and violent social behaviour.*
>
> *The attainment of this target could be significantly supported by developing integrated programmes aimed at reducing the con-sumption of alcohol and other harmful substances by at least 25% by the year 2000.*

The task

Targets 16 and 17 are the two halves of one goal: positive health. Although target 17 arises from the old view of health and target 16 from the new, together they offer immense opportunities for im-proving health and fascinating topics for research.

Lifestyles can be divided into two types according to their effects on health: health-damaging and health-enhancing. Far more is known about the first than the second.

Priority topics

Behaviour that puts health at risk. Scientific evidence on certain types of behaviour warrants classifying them unambiguously as damaging to health. This category includes: smoking, excessive alcohol use, the abuse of therapeutic and mood-altering drugs, inappropriate eating habits and nutritional patterns, lack of physi-cal exercise, dangerous driving and violent behaviour.

The harm that such behaviour can do to health has been thoroughly studied and, at least in principle, generally accepted. Large-scale intervention programmes are needed to reduce them. Research could contribute by:

● analysing the purposes served by these forms of risk behaviour for the people who practise them;

● determining the social forces that tend directly or indirectly to stabilize and encourage such behaviour;

130

- developing, testing and comparing the intervention strategies aimed at both people and social forces; and

- evaluating the resulting intervention programmes.

Many programmes and measures are proposed to reduce the occurrence of health-damaging behaviour. Research could contribute to the achievement of target 17 mainly through a detailed evaluation of the proposed programmes and a comparative analysis of different models for such programmes. The findings would lead to objective assessments of success and failure, and identify both obstacles to successful implementation and the most promising models for effective and efficient programmes. An additional task is the detection of the unintended harmful consequences of health promotion programmes. These could include the encouragement through information campaigns of experimentation with harmful substances or possible victim-blaming as a result of programmes for behavioural change.

Among the types of behaviour that damage health directly, violent social behaviour is obviously one of the most serious problems. The prevalence of organized violence and of violent sexual behaviour (such as child abuse, spouse-beating and rape) is alarmingly high in the European Region. Measures against these types of behaviour call for research into the extent of the problems and into the individual and social causes of violence. Programmes to reduce violent behaviour do not seem to succeed if they tackle the problem in isolation. A better solution seems to be structural changes to reduce inequality in society and much concerted effort in education and health education. These measures would encourage people to feel concern for the health and wellbeing of others. Reducing the occurrence of risk behaviour would certainly improve the health of the general population.

The risk entailed in other forms of behaviour is not yet proven. Both research and health education programmes tend to concentrate on the well known types of risk behaviour, probably because individuals engage in them. Attempts to reduce risks to health can thus be aimed at these people, rather than at social institutions or people in authority. As a result, the concept of risk behaviour is in danger of being narrowed down to misbehaviour.

Launching large-scale intervention programmes on suspected forms of risk behaviour cannot, perhaps, be justified. Enough knowledge is available, however, to justify major research directed at the damage that some widespread behaviour may do to health. Studies should assess such behaviour, which society accepts, imposes or even rewards. Fruitful topics include:

- the patterns of behaviour connected to work (such as chronic stress resulting from excessive time pressure, and social conflicts arising from working conditions, too much ambition, workaholism, shift work, and the relegation of the unemployed to the margins of society);

- the chronic stress resulting from sex-specific role expectations (for example, the double strain on women of filling family and occupational roles and the chronic suppression of emotion often expected of men);

- the risks induced by the health care system (including the making of everyday life into a medical problem, the patient's role as a passive recipient of treatment, and the emphasis on technological aspects of health and health care); and

- the overburdening of people's ability to adapt to rapid social change (such developments as modernization, and the increasing use of computers and demands for occupational mobility).

Long-term interdisciplinary studies will help to single out additional forms of risk behaviour. They will lay the foundation for a fuller understanding of how to reduce the health risks involved. Special attention should be given to looking for the reasons for many types of health-damaging behaviour. Research should investigate the relative impact of individual coping skills, situational stress and a lack of resources on the development and maintenance

132

of harmful practices. For example, people may use mood-altering substances to avoid problems, to reduce feelings of pain or tension caused by problems, to ease social interaction or to attain some form of pleasure and excitement.

Programmes that treat harmful practices as individual behaviour, taking no account of life situation and social environment, are thus unlikely to succeed. The impact of many interacting influences on the formation of lifestyles must be recognized. The development of demonstration projects based on this recognition is therefore a research priority. In addition, mutual-aid groups are an important resource for attempts to change unwanted or damaging behaviour.

Behaviour that improves health. Again, if the positive health approach is to succeed, it must be more clearly defined. Studies must discover how certain lifestyles, or parts of them, benefit health. A good starting point would be research on healthy people, to determine how their behaviour differs from that of others.

So far, research findings point to several aspects of lifestyles that probably help maintain good health. People are more likely to be healthy if they have:

- sufficient income, access to life-long education, and adequate control of working and home life;

- social integration, chances to participate in political, cultural and social life, and sufficient social support in times of crisis;

- a belief that life has purpose and a sense of commitment to others;

- adequate psychological and behavioural mechanisms for coping with problems;

- adequate family planning and sexual wellbeing; and

- self-esteem and feelings of sufficient control over one's own life, health and wellbeing.

133

More intensive research is needed to define positive health. More evidence of the effects of these factors should be collected. In addition, ways of spreading healthy lifestyles should be explored.

A number of programmes and policy actions should promote health through, for example, reducing the manufacture and consumption of tobacco and alcoholic drinks, healthy nutrition, sexual health and family planning, sports and physical activity, and improved coping with stress. Such programmes seem promising. They will succeed, however, only if they can be based on reliable data on patterns of health-related behaviour in various social groups and their effects on health. A decisive prerequisite for both research and programme development is the establishment of a continuously updated data base on lifestyles and their impact on health. More specifically, research is needed to evaluate health promotion programmes and analyse the social obstacles to healthy lifestyles.

Evaluation can support and improve programmes for health promotion. Criteria for judging their effects on behaviour and health should be used whenever possible. Policies should be monitored and assessed for their effects. This would encourage the initiators of programmes to define outcome criteria and to consult experienced scientists in the planning stages. This, in turn, would lead to closer cooperation between research and programme development.

All the objectives mentioned in target 16 are concerned with health education for individuals. People certainly should be encouraged to choose healthy patterns of behaviour. In addition, however, a detailed analysis should be made of the social conditions that promote poor nutrition, smoking and lack of physical activity; and reduce people's ability to cope with stress. At the same time, researchers should explore measures to make health-enhancing behaviour easier to choose and an integral part of everyday life.

For example, researchers should examine structural measures to encourage balanced nutrition. Political and economic analyses of existing taxation and subsidy policies are needed. What are their effects on the production and consumption of various foodstuffs? Such analyses would result in recommendations for taxation and subsidies to support healthy food and dietary patterns. Structural measures on mass catering could affect large groups of people. Descriptive studies could provide information on the nutritional patterns now favoured in this area. Field demonstration projects could explore, test and evaluate alternatives that are healthy, economical and acceptable to consumers.

Research into the sources of stress in work and in other sectors of society should complement the promotion of individuals' ability to cope. Many well established forms of risk behaviour can be considered inappropriate attempts to cope with stress. Any structural measures resulting in a reduction of exposure to chronic stress would therefore tend to reduce health-damaging behaviour and promote health.

6

Health for all in Europe
by the year 2000

Resting on the achievement of the other targets, targets 1–12 detail the improvements in health needed to secure health for all. General goals include equity in health (target 1), the development of health potential (target 2) and better opportunities for the disabled (target 3). Targets 4–12 aim more specifically at reducing the burden of disease and its consequences. While addressing the main chronic, disabling conditions, these nine targets also stress the reduction of premature death due to various causes.

In general, the research recommended for each target is intended to give examples of what could be done in each problem area. Much research on these problems is already under way. This chapter thus emphasizes new research programmes aimed not only at health for all but also at complementing the research programmes in Member States.

Research on all 12 targets must meet five requirements:

- it must address public health needs

- research priorities must be brought up to date;

- the data base must be improved, and internationally accepted indicators must be developed;

**Five requirements
for research**

137

- longitudinal studies and data covering small areas are needed;

- the confidentiality and protection of data must be ensured.

Meeting public health needs

Priority should be given to research projects for the prevention of, treatment for or rehabilitation from the common diseases in each country of the Region. Projects should aim at reducing mortality and morbidity and improving the quality of life. Research objectives should not be restricted to target populations, such as hospital patients, but should extend to morbidity in primary health care and in the community. Therapeutic and evaluative research should concentrate on methods that can be applied effectively in the community and primary care rather than on those that demand the facilities of high-powered modern technology.

Updating research priorities

Targets 1–12 are to be achieved within 12 years. During that time, various kinds of basic and applied research will probably develop rapidly. Advances in molecular biology, biotechnology and computer science may create a need for new research priorities. New techniques for prevention, treatment and rehabilitation may also emerge. For example, progress can be expected in the prevention and treatment of genetic anomalies and of cardiovascular, malignant, rheumatic, psychiatric and other common chronic diseases. In addition, more new viral diseases may appear. Further, new harmful factors in the environment, including psychosocial and economic problems, will pose a variety of threats to people's health. These kinds of change must be taken into account in the monitoring of targets 1–12, and research priorities must be altered accordingly.

More and better information

Taken as a whole, targets 1–12 are a systematic attempt to reduce mortality and morbidity and to improve the quality of life. Setting up a reliable data base is of primary importance in this effort. Data bases will allow the monitoring of changes and progress towards the targets. They should be target-specific, show the links between targets, and be used in intercountry comparisons.

138

Research should determine what data should be collected; how they should be stored, retrieved and analysed; and what kinds of recording system will be needed to monitor specific programmes.

The availability of comparatively reliable statistics on mortality in the Region help to define the targets primarily concerned with fatal diseases. Reduced mortality is thus an indicator of progress, as are data on morbidity and the quality of life. As mortality falls, chronic disabling conditions increase, and the aging of the population augments this trend. Such conditions can be described as the failures of success: the people who suffer from them would previously have died. Progress towards the ambitious goals of the targets will thus be reflected in trends in both the frequency of chronic conditions and in mortality. Such progress must be measured quantitatively.

Research is urgently needed to gather information on: the course and outcome of different forms of health impairment over periods of years, the relevant risk factors, and the effectiveness of different forms of prevention, therapy and rehabilitation. Where adequate data bases already exist, information can be collected retrospectively. In most cases, however, prospective longitudinal studies will be necessary.

Longitudinal studies and small-area data

In addition to more or less well established national health surveys, case registers of different forms of morbidity should be compiled at area level. The information collected should include data on social, economic and other factors relevant to health so that groups at risk can be determined. Data gathered from people interviewed in population-based health surveys are, in general, less reliable than data from health care agencies. The two approaches are, however, complementary.

Health surveys should include data on people's perceptions of their own and their families' health and ability to function, which would provide a more comprehensive idea of health care needs. Area data on needs, preferably collated at community or regional level, are also required to plan programmes and to provide for their evaluation. Models of good practice and care can be best studied at local or community level.

In general, both quantitative and qualitative research will be needed to provide the necessary data. Whenever possible, the findings of studies in different countries should be compared. This means that the same methods and procedures for data collection must be used.

The confidentiality and protection of data

The importance of the confidentiality and protection of data is beyond doubt. Legislation and regulations must not, however, raise unnecessary obstacles to epidemiological and evaluative research. Policy-makers should be alive to the damage that such obstacles may do in the long run to progress in health and to efforts to provide better and more cost-effective care.

Target 1. Equity in health

> *By the year 2000, the actual differences in health status between countries and between groups within countries should be reduced by at least 25%, by improving the level of health of disadvantaged nations and groups.*
>
> *This target could be achieved if the basic prerequisites for health were provided for all; if the risks related to lifestyles were reduced; if the health aspects of living and working conditions were improved; and if good primary health care were made accessible to all.*

The task

Target 1 epitomizes the ultimate goal of the regional strategy for health for all: greater equity in health and health care. Reducing differences in morbidity and mortality among countries and groups within countries is the aim of all the regional targets. Reducing differences in health status by at least 25% is, however, an ambitious goal that may not be realistic for all countries.

Greater equity will be achieved if basic human needs are satisfied. This means, above all, the right kind of food in sufficient quantities, safe drinking-water, good sanitation, and universal,

140

free primary education. People must have: the chance to choose healthy lifestyles (Chapter 5), adequate housing and employment opportunities (in Chapter 4), and good health care (Chapter 3).

In all countries, inequity in health is closely correlated with socioeconomic status. As a result, systematic attempts to improve health standards tend to be based on the simple idea that affluence promotes health and poverty promotes disease. Within certain limits, that assumption holds good. Eradicating severe poverty might be said to be the most important single step towards reducing morbidity. This is, however, an oversimplified view of the problem. Other factors share the responsibility for inequities in health. In some countries, for instance, a woman cannot consult a physician without the consent of her husband. He may refuse because of the cost or because he sees it as a reflection on himself. Children lack equity if they have neglectful or cruel parents. Further, affluence is not a panacea. Some diseases are associated with affluence and are more common among people of higher social status. For example, certain forms of cancer are related to a high-protein diet.

In short, while gross inequities in both health and health care exist in every society, the causes vary, both among and within countries. Inequities may be associated with sex, the underprivileged status accorded to children or old people, immigrant status and other factors, in addition to socioeconomic differences. Measures intended to reduce inequities in health by increasing affluence or improving the quality of life may sometimes increase the incidence of some diseases. Every group in a society has a characteristic pattern of morbidity and mortality, and the more closely groups resemble the one accounted to be privileged, the more they will take on the characteristics of that group. The most striking example of such a trend in Europe is the emancipation of women, which has been associated with an increase in some causes of morbidity and mortality among women (such as lung cancer and suicide) and a reduction in others.

Progress towards greater equity in health obviously requires better data and more reliable indicators on the population. They will ensure that any important trends in morbidity — favourable or unfavourable — can be immediately perceived and assessed. This necessitates the improvement of official statistics and the standard of routine documentation in Member States, and the study of the many causes of inequity in health. Such studies will need standard indicators and research designs to allow international collaboration and ensure the comparability of findings.

Priority topics   *Improving official health statistics.*   To monitor progress towards equity in health, countries must routinely collect data on health differences. Such secondary data must be collated at country, regional and community levels. This will allow comparisons of the health of groups within a population and in different regions. Deficiencies in health can be estimated and priorities for overcoming them set.

The scope of the statistical returns will depend largely on the extent of routine documentation in each country. Whenever possible, countries should try to complement existing statistics on morbidity and mortality with data relevant to inequities in health, covering, for example:

- socioeconomic status (including income, housing conditions, unemployment and underemployment);

- age (with particular emphasis on the problems of the young and the old);

- ethnic and religious differences;

- types of environment (urban or rural) and lifestyle;

- occupational hazards; and

- the availability of health care and related services.

Reliable and, preferably, internationally accepted indicators must be used to compile good health statistics. Continuing the

142

development of reliable and practical regional indicators is a research priority. The indicators should be used to assess inequities in health and make national statistics internationally comparable. WHO should promote this work.

Causes of inequity in health. The many causes of inequities in health are not well understood. Investigating them requires specific studies to obtain primary data. Socioepidemiological research should point out the factors associated with variations in morbidity and mortality among different groups of people. Studies must examine the socioeconomic and other factors that determine health status, and should specify:

- available indicators of health status;

- the extent (and indicators) of social inequities related to health;

- how poverty, bad housing and working conditions, unhealthy patterns of behaviour, and other environmental factors can harm health;

- to what extent lack of equity in health is due to socioeconomic differences, to family lifestyles or to the structure and practices of health care systems;

- the different kinds of health and social services available, where they are available and the extent of their use;

- the strategies, policies or social processes used to reduce social inequities and differences in health status; and

- the policies, types of behaviour or social processes that actually increase social morbidity or hinder prompt and effective health care, and thus tend to worsen health in some groups of people.

Whenever feasible, international collaborative studies should be made on inequities in health. Research in different countries must therefore follow some common guidelines. As far as possible, researchers should use the same indicators, and study designs and methods that will produce comparable findings. Standard methods, even if difficult to achieve, are essential. In this area, WHO can play a decisive role in initiating and promoting the necessary research.

**Target 2.
Adding life to years**

> *By the year 2000, people should have the basic opportunity to develop and use their health potential to live socially and economically fulfilling lives.*
>
> *This target could be achieved if health policies in Member States gave a framework for developing, implementing and monitoring programmes that provide the environmental conditions, social support and services required to develop and use each person's health potential.*

The task

The basis of this target is the idea that everyone should have the chance to live as fulfilling and healthy a life as possible. All people should realize their potential for health as fully as they can.

The general policies for achieving target 2 call for the provision of a healthy environment, social support, and social and health services. All of these encourage people to maintain good health, and special importance is given to solving the problems of the elderly. These general activities were discussed in Chapters 3–5. The discussion of target 2 concentrates on needs for research on specific measures, including those for the benefit of children and young people.

Priority topics

Developing indicators of positive health.   WHO stresses that both society and the individual are responsible for developing health potential. Indicators of positive health should be used to monitor progress towards target 2. This requires, above all, a clearer concept of positive health. Research on health indicators and on social psychiatry and rehabilitation has developed and refined measures of functional status and quality of life. These measures provide an approach to research on positive health.

Again, people's own perceptions of their health must be taken into account in evaluations of health care. Self-assessment measures have already been developed and used successfully in addition to objective ratings. Some evidence indicates that they are especially useful in evaluating positive health.

Researchers should begin or continue to define what is meant by a state of physical, mental and social wellbeing, and its biological and genetic components. Indicators of positive health are needed to evaluate productive life as an element of self-fulfilment for working people. Such indicators could also determine the effectiveness of rehabilitation programmes.

Early detection of retardation. Children and young people are the most important target groups in any endeavour to develop health potential. Systematic health promotion should start as early as possible in life.

Early detection of intellectual and developmental retardation is an important first step towards:

- reducing subsequent handicaps to a minimum;

- determining risk factors before, during and after birth, or in early life; and

- evaluating the effectiveness of such preventive measures as immunization programmes.

Research should determine the incidence of intellectual and developmental retardation among preschool children. How is it associated with known risk factors in pregnancy, at birth and after birth? What specific preventive measures could be taken during these periods? Studies should take account of environmental factors that may be relevant, including family and socioeconomic variables in both industrial and rural areas. The nutrition of babies and small children must also receive particular attention. Studies should include systematic screening and surveillance of risk and control groups of children during their preschool years. The samples or cohorts of children should be drawn from the general population. Support programmes for the affected children should be carefully evaluated.

Problems of elderly people.   The obstacles to communication and interaction between generations are an important topic in evaluating the problems of the elderly. In addition, studies should evaluate education programmes that emphasize opportunities for aging people to maintain their own health. Research should assess the importance of systematic preparation for retirement and of opportunities for useful and enjoyable activities in retirement.

The effects of retirement on physical and mental health should also be examined. The results of enforced or officially encouraged early retirement should be compared with those of flexible, phased approaches. Finally, research should determine the social, cultural, economic, genetic, physical and lifestyle factors that make for a successful adaptation to aging.

Target 3.
Better opportunities
for the disabled

> *By the year 2000, disabled persons should have the physical, social and economic opportunities that allow at least for a socially and economically fulfilling and mentally creative life.*
>
> *This target could be achieved if societies developed positive attitudes towards the disabled and set up programmes aimed at providing appropriate physical, social and economic opportunities for them to develop their capacities to lead a healthy life.*

The task   Social integration is a general aim in attempts to offer better opportunities to the disabled. This entails preventing the exclusion

146

or segregation of disabled people from society, enabling them to lead normal social lives within the limits imposed by their conditions, and encouraging them to remain with their families or in their communities as long as possible. Better social integration of the disabled will, in turn, help other people to develop positive attitudes towards them.

The principle of normalization applies to such widely different target groups as the young chronically sick, the mentally retarded, and elderly people who are physically and mentally impaired. It must be included in research into the merits of different forms of care and the best ways of assessing their effectivness.

Two forms of care for the disabled. The merits of institutional and community-based care should be compared. Research should determine the extent to which adequate care can be provided by agencies in the community, and the most appropriate and effective forms of long-term care for disabled people who cannot remain in the community. Reliable indicators of the quality and the effectiveness of care, and of the attitudes of society to the disabled, are essential in all investigations. Studies of both kinds of care should begin with reviews of research on these subjects in the European Region. Developments in various countries can thus be compared. The cost-effectiveness of various technical aids to allow the disabled to care for themselves should also be assessed.

The effectiveness of rehabilitation. Indicators of the effectiveness of rehabilitation or supportive programmes for the chronically disabled are more and more necessary. These measures should not rely exclusively on working capacity or reintegration into the labour force. They should measure people's ability to fulfil their daily tasks (even if these are unpaid), their social adjustment, leisure activities and other kinds of self-fulfilment. Such indicators are particularly important in studies of disabled housewives, the elderly, the unemployed and other people who do not hold paid jobs.

Priority topics

147

> *By the year 2000, the average number of years that people live free from major disease and disability should be increased by at least 10%.*
>
> *This target could be achieved if, for instance, comprehensive programmes aimed at primary prevention of accidents and violence, cardiovascular disease, lifestyle-related cancers, occupational diseases, psychiatric disorders, alcoholism and drug abuse were developed, and adequate curative and rehabilitative services provided to all; if current knowledge regarding infectious diseases prevention were systematically applied; if genetic counselling services were made more generally available; if research were intensified with regard to disabling neurological and musculoskeletal disorders; and if preventive measures in oral health were effectively implemented.*

The task

This target and those that follow concentrate on combating certain major threats to health. The discussion of target 4 focuses on: tackling infectious diseases that are of special importance to the Region or particularly difficult to control (such as AIDS), and reducing disability from genetic conditions and congenital anomalies, mental illness, rheumatic conditions, and caries and periodontal disease. Disability resulting from preventable infectious diseases (target 5), cardiovascular diseases (target 9), cancer (target 10), accidents (target 11) and occupational diseases (target 25, Chapter 6) is dealt with elsewhere.

Priority topics

Infectious diseases. Research into the immunology and virology of AIDS should be strenuously promoted. Epidemiological studies on people with AIDS and those who have human immunodeficiency virus (HIV) are required, as well as research into the psychosocial and economic aspects of the problem. Member States should develop educational programmes for health personnel and the general public to prevent or limit the spread of HIV. These programmes should be monitored for effectiveness.

In addition, research should focus in general on the production of new vaccines for diseases caused by viruses, including retroviruses. Viruses that contribute to disease (such as human papilloma viruses 16 and 18 in cervical cancer, EB virus and nasopharyngeal cancer and hepatitis virus B) should also be included.

Attention should also be paid to infectious diseases with late sequelae. These include acute respiratory and urinary infections and sexually transmitted diseases resulting in infertility. Research and epidemiological surveys on prevention are required if further progress is to be made.

Genetic conditions and congenital anomalies. The effectiveness of prenatal and neonatal screening for genetic conditions and congenital anomalies is not well established; more research is needed on such programmes. How should they be applied? Who should be screened and how? What are the legal and ethical issues? What psychological and social impact do they make on the family? Are screening programmes accepted by the population? How widely available are genetic counselling services in the European Region?

Further, there is evidence that genetic factors play a part in several of the most common health problems, such as coronary heart disease. DNA research, focusing on genetic conditions and congenital anomalies, is a new, exciting field of basic research that requires further exploration. It could contribute to better diagnosis and better knowledge of the etiology of disease.

Basic research on DNA, however, is a highly specialized form of scientific inquiry. It must be carried out in centres with the requisite equipment and staff. The findings can then be made available to all countries so that the research is not replicated elsewhere. Moreover, careful attention should be paid to the possibility that such research may have unintended consequences. Research programmes should be monitored with that possibility in mind.

Mental health problems. In many European countries, the most pressing problems in mental health arise from the aging of the population and the high incidence of alcohol and drug abuse.

Little information is available about the incidence of specific categories of mental disorder in the elderly (such as senile dementia and multi-infarct dementia) and their relationship to various risk factors. Epidemiological research into these questions is urgently required. It poses a number of methodological problems, however, that must be resolved before valid findings can be obtained. Simple, reliable methods of assessing cognitive impairment are needed. They could be applied in case-finding, especially in primary health care, for earlier detection, diagnosis and treatment. Depression is common in the elderly; its prognosis is often relatively poor. More intensive and systematic studies should determine the factors that influence the course and outcome of late-life depressive states. Research should also discover the scope for more effective treatment and care.

Reliable, objective measures are also needed of the severity of abuse of and dependence on alcohol and drugs. Systematic studies in both clinical settings and the community should establish how and to what extent patterns of dependence and abuse depend on the substance in question, on personal characterics and on the social environment. Scientists should search for biochemical or other markers for use in screening or monitoring for the abuse of alcohol and other psychoactive substances. Such methods could be applied in testing for associations between certain health and social problems and substance abuse in individuals and groups. To satisfy ethical requirements, screening should only be done with the informed consent of the subjects and careful regard for the confidentiality of the results.

Research is also urgently needed to determine the extent and nature of the relationships between various types of drug dependence and psychiatric disorders in middle and late life, such as schizophrenia, affective disorders and organic mental syndromes. Whenever possible, this research should be designed to include non-patient or non-institutional populations. Investigations should

150

determine whether or how people with compulsive patterns of substance abuse differ from others who use these substances heavily or habitually without losing control.

Rheumatic disease. Better epidemiological surveys are needed on the prevalence and incidence of rheumatic conditions in the population. Special attention should be paid to the degenerative diseases and diseases of the connective tissue.

Studies should concentrate on discovering predisposing factors and preventive measures. More vigorous research is required to establish the relationship between degenerative rheumatic conditions and physical activity, nutrition, and psychological, immunological, genetic, socioeconomic, occupational and other risk factors. Such results could lead to effective means of prevention, including healthy lifestyles.

More effective methods of treatment, care and rehabilitation are required to prevent chronicity and deterioration in rheumatic disease. Both pain-relieving treatment and physical and social rehabilitation services in the community need to be systematically evaluated.

Oral disease. Programmes to prevent oral disease, the reduction of risk factors and the regular intake of fluoride are important in reducing caries and periodontal disease. Educational programmes including oral hygiene should begin early in people's lives and secondary caries prevention at school age should be encouraged. Preventive programmes must be monitored for effectiveness.

Research into the oral health of the elderly and into the provision of oral health care for the elderly should be encouraged.

The fluoridation of drinking-water, although effective in preventing caries, is not always feasible or acceptable. Nor can it replace a healthy diet. A nutrition policy designed to control caries (and including the reduction of the sugar content of sweets and other types of food) requires further exploration. It also has wider implications for health promotion.

**Target 5.
Eliminating
seven specific diseases**

> *By the year 2000, there should be no indigenous measles, polio-myelitis, neonatal tetanus, congenital rubella, diphtheria, congenital syphilis or indigenous malaria in the Region.*
>
> *This target could be achieved through a well organized primary health care system ensuring effective epidemiological surveillance, vaccination coverage, malaria control measures, education on the risks of syphilis, screening and, when necessary, treatment of expectant mothers.*

Priority topics

The conditions specified in this target are mainly preventable. In general, they can be controlled through vaccination, but both controlling and eliminating them pose logistical problems. In some countries, immunization and control programmes for these diseases are still inadequate and eradication is far away; neonatal tetanus and poliomyelitis are two examples that deserve further research. It is important to examine the reasons why such preventable conditions have not yet disappeared from the European Region.

**Target 6.
Life expectancy
at birth**

> *By the year 2000, life expectancy at birth in the Region should be at least 75 years.*
>
> *This target could be achieved if, by the year 2000, no country or group within a country had a life expectancy of less than 65 years; if countries that reached this level in 1980 had a life expectancy of more than 75 years; and if all countries had reduced by at least 25% the differences in life expectancy among geographical areas and socioeconomic groups and between the sexes.*

Priority topics

Because greater life expectancy means reduced mortality, this target can be seen as an introduction to targets 7–12, which deal

152

with combating some of the most important causes of death in order to increase life expectancy at birth substantially.

The reduction of specific causes of mortality, however, may not by itself substantially diminish the differences in life expectancy between geographical areas, socioeconomic groups and the sexes. No single diagnosis is likely to explain the overall differences. The general factors underlying the differences in levels of health must also be investigated.

By the year 2000, infant mortality in the Region should be less than 20 per 1000 live births.   *This target could be achieved if, by the year 2000, no country or group within a country had an infant mortality rate of more than 40 per 1000 live births; if countries with a rate below this level in 1980 had a rate below 15 per 1000; and if all countries attempted to reduce significantly the differences among geographical areas and socioeconomic groups.*

**Target 7.
Reducing
infant mortality rates**

By the year 2000, maternal mortality in the Region should be less than 15 per 100 000 live births.   *This target could be achieved if, by the year 2000, no country or group within a country had a maternal mortality rate of more than 25 per 100 000 live births; if countries with a rate already below 25 in 1980 had a rate below 10; and if all countries had reduced significant differences among geographical areas and socioeconomic groups.*

**Target 8.
Reducing rates
of maternal mortality**

These two targets will be discussed together because they present closely interrelated problems. Rates of infant and maternal mortality in the Region are already low. Today, the reduction of

The task

153

morbidity in infants and mothers has higher priority in most countries than further reductions in mortality. The recommendations for research therefore deal with both goals.

Sudden infant death syndrome.   The sudden infant death syndrome is one of the major causes of infant mortality. Epidemiological surveys are needed to establish the magnitude and distribution of this problem and its associated risk factors.

Variations in infant and maternal mortality.   Some of the causes of the relatively high rates of infant and maternal mortality in developing parts of the European Region are well known. The direct causes of the large variations in mortality among socioeconomic groups should be further investigated.

Perinatal technology.   Most Member States have seen a rapid proliferation of new perinatal technology, such as *in vitro* fertilization. Few of these machines, drugs and procedures have been adequately evaluated for their benefits, hazards, effectiveness, cost, ethics and social impact. Perinatal technology needs careful scientific scrutiny. Health services research should examine the various aspects of care given before, during and after birth. The attitudes and perceptions of the users of the services should be included in the assessments.

Key issues for research include:

- the relative merits and safety of high-technology as opposed to low-technology services for both mother and baby;

- the cost–benefit ratio of an interventionist approach in obstetrics;

- the ethical and social impact of high technology on birth; and

- models of good practice in perinatal care.

Low birth weight.   More research into the causes of low birth weight would help prevent infant mortality and morbidity. Studies should focus on the effects of nutrition, smoking and drinking during pregnancy, and on environmental, social and genetic factors. These have attracted much recent interest in twin, family and adoption research.

Breastfeeding. Evidence of the beneficial effects of breastfeeding — on infant survival, child growth and development and in the prevention of infant morbidity — continues to accumulate. The factors that militate against breastfeeding need to be determined. Those affecting young, poor and less educated mothers are particularly important as such women seem less likely to breastfeed. Methods of marketing and selling breast-milk substitutes, particularly to these women, should be carefully monitored and scrutinized.

Monitoring morbidity and mortality. To attain targets 7 and 8, groups of women known to be at risk — the socially disadvantaged, immigrants and the very young — must not only have access to but actually use available services, such as family planning services, perinatal care, and support services. The monitoring and analysis of variations in infant and maternal mortality and morbidity among countries and groups within countries should show whether or how programmes for these risk groups have succeeded.

By the year 2000, mortality in the Region from diseases of the circulatory system in people under 65 should be reduced by at least 15%.

This target could be achieved by a combination of preventive and treatment methods that would reverse the trend in countries where ischaemic heart disease mortality is increasing or stable, and accelerate it in countries where the mortality is decreasing, thereby contributing to the current decline in cerebrovascular mortality in all countries.

**Target 9.
Combating diseases
of the circulatory system**

The task   A combination of prevention and treatment methods, including rehabilitation, is needed to reduce the number of deaths from diseases of the circulatory system. Although the aim of this target applies to all age groups, mortality among people under 65 years of age can be a convenient indicator for monitoring progress in a way that is relatively independent of differences in age distribution between different populations.

Priority topics   *Evaluating preventive measures and reducing risk factors.*   The major risk factors in cardiovascular diseases (smoking, high blood pressure and raised blood cholesterol) are well established, although their predictive power is limited. Additional risk factors (including psychosocial risks) and their interaction with those already known require study. Further research is also needed into the problems of controlling hypertension: monitoring trends in blood pressure, developing and testing methods of treatment that do not include drugs, and finding better methods of prevention, such as health education.

Reducing the major risk factors in cardiovascular diseases requires preventive measures at community level, starting in childhood. Programmes can aim, for example, at discouraging smoking, promoting a healthy diet, reducing obesity, controlling blood pressure and reducing aggressive competitive behaviour in professional life. These programmes need careful evaluation. Studies of antismoking campaigns, for example, should analyse the reasons for failure and find out how to involve the mass media in campaigns with alternative approaches to preventing cardiovascular diseases. Programmes should be aimed at high-risk groups, as well as at the general population.

Improving treatment and rehabilitation.   Treatment and rehabilitation programmes are needed to improve the prognosis and reduce the risk of repeat acute myocardial infarction and stroke. The available knowledge on nutritional and other factors that affect prognosis, including psychological and educational elements, can

156

be used in the planning of programmes. In addition, such programmes must be monitored for effectiveness and for acceptance by patients.

Using genetic research. The use of results from genetic research may accelerate progress in combating cardiovascular diseases. Evidence of the contribution of genetic factors to mortality from circulatory diseases (especially in men under 55 years of age and women under 60) is almost irrefutable. The total population approach used in previous studies of risk factors and interventions has tended to ignore individual predisposition to coronary heart disease.

Studies must investigate the role of genetic, environmental and nutritional risk factors. Social stress and combinations of risk factors should be examined, as well as protective factors. The idea that environmental and nutritional factors cause coronary heart disease mainly in people genetically predisposed to it will permit more effective and specific disease control as soon as predictive testing can be performed.

Research is needed into predictive testing, especially by DNA technology. Again, basic DNA research cannot be an integral part of country research for health for all. Nevertheless, the findings of such research may in future be used to control disease and thus contribute to health for all.

By the year 2000, mortality in the Region from cancer in people under 65 should be reduced by at least 15%.	**Target 10.** **Combating cancer**

This target could be achieved if tobacco-related cancers were reduced as a result of a major decrease in smoking and cervical cancer following the establishment of screening programmes; and if current methods in early diagnosis, treatment and rehabilitation were applied in an appropriate way to all cancer patients.

The task   While the aim of this target — reducing mortality from cancer — applies to all age groups, mortality among people under 65 years of age may be a convenient indicator of success. This must not be taken to mean, however, that therapeutic or preventive programmes should not cover people older than 65.

A variety of actions will attain the target. These include:

- a reduction in smoking (see target 16, Chapter 5);

- multidisciplinary research into nutritional, reproductive, infective or other factors in cancer;

- the limitation of occupational exposure to asbestos and air pollution (see Chapter 4), the unnecessary use of X-rays and certain drugs in health care, and overexposure of the skin to sunlight;

- the use of screening for early detection of cancer of the cervix and the breast; and

- better diagnosis and treatment for cancer, based on the results of scientific research.

Priority topics   The studies of antismoking campaigns recommended under target 9 would be equally useful for fighting cancer. The other topics recommended are either important in the health for all programme or may become so in the near future.

Multidisciplinary research into risks.   Needs for knowledge on the role of viruses in cancer etiology were mentioned in the discussion of target 5. The relationship of nutrition to cancer risks also deserves higher research priority. Evidence shows that dietary patterns are important in the etiology of some types of cancer. The consumption of foods rich in fibre and vitamins and low in fat (fresh fruit and vegetables) seems to be associated with a low incidence of cancer, although this connection is not yet clearly established. The possibilities of preventing cancer through nutritional measures have not yet been studied.

158

Screening for early detection.   More and more evidence shows that countrywide screening could reduce mortality through the early detection of cancer of the cervix and breast. Screening programmes should include standards for the treatment of women with detected cancers. The cost–benefit ratios of such programmes must also be carefully monitored.

The reasons for delays in diagnosis and treatment should be determined as a part of evaluative studies. Delay on the part of the patient may be an important indicator of deficiencies in health education; people must know that cancer is often preventable and can often be treated successfully when it occurs. Similarly, delay on the part of the health professional may point to deficiencies in the health services.

Existing screening programmes should be extended to visible types of cancer, such as oral and skin cancer. The results of the programmes should be evaluated for the numbers of cases detected and the benefit to the affected people. Research is also required to develop and evaluate methods for the early detection of gastrointestinal tumours.

Research on diagnosis, treatment and rehabilitation.   Special priority should be given to health services research to improve the use of existing knowledge in the health care system. Important subjects include the assessment of the technology used in cancer control and care (see target 38, Chapter 2), with special emphasis on: the quality of life of people with cancer; the use of electronic data processing to organize population-based screening, surveillance, recall and follow-up; continuity of care for people with cancer detected through screening; and the merits of routine screening for oral cancer during visits to the dentist.

New methods of preventing, diagnosing and treating cancer are expected to result from progress in molecular biology. Research in this area is increasing rapidly. More research is also needed to improve the care of people with cancer. Dealing with the psychosocial problems of patients and their families is particularly important. Evaluative research can help to improve standards of care and point out the most effective and useful components of programmes.

**Target 11.
Reducing accidents**

By the year 2000, deaths from accidents in the Region should be reduced by at least 25% through an intensified effort to reduce traffic, home and occupational accidents.

This target could be achieved if, by the year 2000, no country had a mortality rate from road traffic accidents of more than 20 per 100 000; if countries below that level reduced it to less than 15; if all countries reduced the differences between the sexes, and age and socioeconomic groups; furthermore, if the occupational accident mortality in the Region were lowered by at least 50%; and if the mortality from home accidents were significantly reduced.

The task

Research is needed to overcome obstacles to the application of existing knowledge and to improve the information routinely available, in order to establish better prevention and intervention programmes. Detailed information, specific for place and country, is lacking on the epidemiology of accidents and on existing programmes of prevention and control. Many measures are based on false assumptions because of ignorance in these areas.

Priority topics

Obstacles to the use of existing knowledge. Accidents, particularly traffic and occupational accidents, could be substantially reduced if the knowledge available were fully used. High priority should be given to investigations of the major political, social, economic and psychological obstacles to using this knowledge to reduce accident risks.

Improving informaiton on accidents and preventive measures. The system of information on accidents has several gaps and shortcomings. Statistics often include the causes — such as poisoning — but do not precisely identify the sites of accidents, other than those

160

involving motor vehicles or occurring at work. Although most accidents seem to take place in the home, the damage to health is difficult to assess. The health services report only the small proportion of accidents resulting in death. One important line of research is the associations between serious risk in children and psychological problems in the family, such as depression in the mother.

A more comprehensive information system would permit epidemiological studies of the circumstances of accidents, the role of personal and environmental risk factors, and the effectiveness of specific or general measures for prevention. Evidence from a number of countries shows that, for instance, the rate of traffic accidents is related to alcohol consumption and to the frequency of alcohol abuse. Studies have also indicated that the use of psychoactive drugs is a significant factor. Epidemiological studies should determine the links between the use of alcohol or drugs and road accidents. They should also monitor the effects on the accident rate of measures aimed at reducing the abuse of alcohol, drugs and psychoactive substances.

Standard indicators and assessment methods are needed to ensure that the findings of these studies are internationally comparable.

Monitoring safety measures. Safety measures include traffic control and safety education for road users, the improvement of machinery and roads, child-proof containers for medicines, building and fire codes, and the control of occupational hazards. The protective effects of such measures need careful monitoring. The level of individual compliance with safety regulations should also be investigated.

Many countries in the Region do not yet have comprehensive safety codes. Research should therefore seek to establish the relationship between the frequency of accidents and the existence and enforcement of such codes.

Preventing and dealing with accidents. Safety measures to prevent accidents occurring at home and at play deserve particular

161

attention. Intervention programmes must be based on more accurate knowledge of the causes of such accidents and of the people most at risk: children and the elderly. Research into preventing falls and fractures in the elderly is of high priority.

The effects of imposing maximum speed limits on road traffic need to be impartially evaluated through systematic research and the monitoring of traffic accidents.

As people often take risks deliberately, research should also seek ways to turn such behaviour into less dangerous channels.

Research must also be involved in improving the system of surveillance of, contingency planning for, and response to major accidents and disasters. For example, studies should investigate the most cost-effective ways of setting up emergency services or adapting and improving existing services to deal with such contingencies.

Target 12. Stopping the increase in suicides

> *By the year 2000, the current rising trends in suicides and attempted suicides in the Region should be reversed.*
>
> *This target could be achieved if improvements were made with regard to societal factors that put a strain on the individual, such as unemployment and social isolation; if the individual's ability to cope with life events were strengthened by education and social support; and if the health and social service personnel were better trained to deal with people at high risk.*

The task

The numbers of suicides in the majority of European countries have increased considerably in both sexes and almost all age groups. In general, the incidence of suicide has tended to increase with age, the highest rates being found among people aged 65 years and more. A second peak, however, in the group aged 45–54 has begun to appear. Further, significant trends have been noted among men aged 15–44 years and among women aged 25–44 and 65–74.

162

Rates of suicide are generally low among children and young people but recently have turned upwards. The relationship of such suicides to family, school and social problems, and the effectiveness of preventive measures are now important subjects for study.

The prevention of suicide should not be seen as an isolated objective, but as one of the major goals of programmes aimed at improving people's health. Preventive approaches must try to ensure an acceptable quality of life for all citizens, including people suffering from incurable disease or chronic illness and disability. All research to develop more or less specific measures to prevent suicide should be seen in this broader perspective.

Research can help to attain this target through: work on better methods of documenting suicide and attempted suicide, the evaluation of preventive programmes, and studies on high-risk groups.

Better methods of documentation.   Any systematic attempt to halt or reverse current trends in rates of suicide and attempted suicide must depend on effective, reliable methods of documenting these events. The information should be recorded in a way that allows it to be used for monitoring and to provide guidance for the planning and development of preventive measures.

Priority topics

Suicide and attempted suicide are different phenomena, affecting different risk groups, with different medical and social correlates. To a large extent, they should be dealt with separately. Suicide statistics must generally be collated at national or federal level, while statistics on attempted suicide can be most reliably collated in selected areas with defined populations and served by local hospitals and community agencies. It is important to distinguish between rates for the general public or patients, for episodes and for first-ever and repeated attempts.

Evaluation of preventive programmes.   No planned, systematic programmes of prevention have so far been shown to be effective. All programmes, therefore, must be regarded as experimental and subjected to careful evaluation. Given the present lack of

163

knowledge of effective methods of preventing suicide, case control studies in this field are ethically justifiable and scientifically necessary.

The effects of modified practices in prescribing hypnosedatives and other potentially harmful drugs should be systematically studied.

Studies of high-risk groups.   The most promising lines of inquiry in suicide prevention point to determining and, if possible, helping the groups in the population known to be at high risk. These include: people suffering from severe depression, people dependent on alcohol or drugs, middle-aged and elderly people who have been socially isolated by changed family and social circumstances, and people who have already made one or more serious suicide attempts.

More systematic methods of case-finding are required. The effectiveness of personnel in general practice, other primary health care services, and social agencies in recognizing people at risk of suicide should be assessed. Experimental methods for improving case detection should be tested.

Studies should be directed not only at groups of people but also at the populations of certain defined areas, particularly inner-city areas known to have high rates of social isolation, unemployment and social pathology. Rates of unemployment in many countries remain high, and unemployment and suicidal behaviour are known to be associated. Research on such behaviour among jobless people and in areas with high or rapidly increasing unemployment should therefore be given high priority.

In all studies of people at risk, it will be important to obtain information on successive population cohorts. This is the only way to distinguish changes in suicide risk from other secular effects, such as changes in the age structure of populations and in age-related factors such as unemployment.